Chair Tai Chi for Weight Loss

A Seated Workout Guide for Seniors to Lose Weight, Build Strength, and Boost Mobility — Safe 28-Day Exercise Program, 10 Mins a Day, No Standing Required

Jing Weston

Disclaimer

The content in this book is provided for educational purposes and general guidance only. Nothing here replaces a consultation with your doctor or a qualified medical professional. Before starting this seated program or any new form of physical activity, please speak with your physician, especially if you are managing a chronic condition, recovering from injury or surgery, or have recently been unwell.

The author and publisher have taken care to present this material responsibly. Even so, neither accepts liability for any adverse outcome, injury, or loss that may arise from following the guidance in these pages. Use your own judgment, listen to your body, and consult a professional when in doubt.

Table of Contents

A Note from the Author

Somewhere along the way, the chair got a bad reputation in wellness conversations. It became shorthand for what people were trying to move away from, the thing you sat in when you were not doing something useful for your body. Get up from the chair. Get moving. Stop sitting so much.

I understand where that comes from. Prolonged, passive sitting, the kind where nothing in the body is engaged, where hours pass without any deliberate movement, does real physiological harm. That is documented and true. But the chair itself is not the problem. What you do in it, and whether you ever approach it with any intention at all, is the thing that matters.

This book is built on a simple idea: that the chair can be the beginning of a movement practice, not the end of one. That ten minutes of seated Tai Chi, done every day, produces genuine physiological changes. That you do not have to stand up to lose weight, build functional strength, or improve how your body moves through the world.

I have worked with people in their sixties, seventies, and eighties who came to me because standing exercise was no longer possible or safe for them. Some had significant joint problems. Some had balance conditions. Some had simply reached a point where the risk of a fall outweighed whatever benefit a standing workout might offer. These were not people who had given up. They were people who needed a different starting point.

What I found, working with them, was that seated Tai Chi produced results I had not fully anticipated. Improved energy, reduced morning stiffness, better sleep, a quieter nervous system, and, over time, changes in body composition. Not dramatic, not overnight. But consistent and real. The mechanisms behind these changes are the same whether the practitioner is standing or seated: cortisol reduction through diaphragmatic breathing, muscle activation through sustained controlled movement, circulation improvement through deliberate whole-body engagement. The chair changes the platform. It does not change the physiology.

This program asks ten minutes of your day. Not ten strenuous minutes. Ten deliberate ones. You will learn eight seated forms from the Tai Chi tradition, adapted specifically for chair practice. You will learn a breathing technique that begins working on cortisol from the first session. You will follow a 28-day structure that builds one week at a time, adding forms and increasing duration gradually so the body adapts rather than resists.

I want to be direct about expectations. You are not going to transform your body in 28 days. Nobody will promise you that here. What you will likely notice, often within the first week, is something more immediate: your mornings feel slightly different. The stiffness in your hips or lower back resolves a little faster. You sit more easily for longer. Your energy in the mid-morning, which may have been unreliable for years, begins to steady. These are real changes. They precede the changes that show up on a scale, and they are more reliably produced than scale changes are.

Read through the first two chapters before you begin the program. They explain why the practice works at a physiological level, and that understanding tends to keep people practicing on the mornings when motivation is thin. Then read Chapter Three, which sets up your practice space and teaches you the one thing that matters before any form begins: how to sit with intention.

The chair is not a limitation. It is where we start. Every form in this book begins from a chair. Every breath begins from a chair. Every session ends in one. And over the course of 28 days of consistent practice, the chair becomes not a place of passivity but of genuine, deliberate, productive work.

That is what I want for you. Let's begin.

Jing Weston

Before You Begin

A few things to take care of before the first session. None of this takes long, but each one matters, done properly, they will make every session that follows feel steadier and more effective.

Medical Disclaimer

Please consult your doctor before beginning this program. This applies particularly if you have cardiovascular disease, diabetes, severe osteoporosis, a recent joint replacement or surgery, significant balance impairment, or any condition your doctor actively monitors. A good physician will help you modify where needed rather than simply say no, and there is almost always a modification available.

The movements in this book are all performed seated and are among the lowest-impact forms of exercise available. The program is designed for people who prefer or require seated exercise for any reason. Still, individual responses vary. If any movement causes sharp pain, dizziness, shortness of breath, or significant discomfort, stop immediately. Try again tomorrow with a reduced range of motion, or consult a professional who can observe you directly.

Mild discomfort that eases as the body warms up is different from pain. Most people over sixty carry some stiffness in the morning and some residual tension in the hips, lower back, and shoulders. The forms in this book address all of those areas. What they should never cause is the kind of sharp, localized, worsening pain that signals something is wrong. That distinction matters and only you can make it.

This book is educational material, not medical treatment. The author and publisher accept no liability for any injury or outcome. Your health decisions are your own.

What You Need

One sturdy chair. This is the only equipment this program requires. The chair must be armless so your arms can move freely through the full range of each form. It must have a firm, level seat, not a soft cushion that your pelvis sinks into. The seat height should allow your feet to rest flat on the floor with your knees at approximately a right angle. A standard dining or kitchen chair is usually ideal.

The chair must not roll or wobble. Stability is not negotiable. If the chair you have slides on a hard floor, place a non-slip mat under it or practice on carpet.

Comfortable clothing that does not restrict at the shoulders or hips. Loose trousers, a comfortable top. Nothing tight across the upper back or arms, since several of the forms use full shoulder rotation.

Flat shoes or bare feet. The forms are seated, so footwear is less critical than in standing Tai Chi. What matters is that your feet can rest flat on the floor and make stable contact with it. Shoes with very thick soles can reduce this contact.

Somewhere reasonably quiet, if you can manage it. The early sessions are easier when you can give the forms your full attention without fighting background noise. That said, occasional sound is fine, what disrupts practice is not noise so much as constant interruption that breaks the session apart.

That is the complete list. No mat, no resistance bands, no apps, no equipment purchases. The chair is the practice space.

One additional note: if pain or discomfort in a specific joint affects your ability to perform certain arm or hip movements, note which movements those are before you start. Every form in Chapter Four includes an IF NEEDED modification that reduces range of motion or changes the movement pattern. You will not need to skip anything entirely. You will need to know where your current limits are so you can work within them safely.

How to Use This Book

Start wherever your instincts lead you. If you are someone who likes to understand what you are doing before you do it, begin at Chapter One. It explains the physiology behind seated movement in plain terms, why ten minutes from a chair can do what it does, and what is actually happening inside the body when you practice.

If you would rather start moving and read later, go straight to Chapter Three. It sets up your chair, your posture, and the breathing technique that runs through every session, and the self-assessment you will return to during the progress checks in Chapter Five. Read Chapter Three before Day 1.

Chapter Four is the movement library. All eight seated forms, written out in full with step-by-step instructions. When Chapter Five (the 28-day program) tells you which forms to do each day, Chapter Four is where you find the details. Chapters Six through Eight cover nutrition, between-session movement, and what to do once the 28 days are over. Read them when you are ready.

fReady to begin without reading further? Chapter Three sets up your practice. Chapter Four walks you through all eight forms. Then open Chapter Five and find Day 1. If you prefer to read through the whole book first, that works just as well, start here and follow it through.

Chapter 1

Yes, You Can Lose Weight Sitting Down

The title of this chapter is a claim, and claims require evidence. This chapter provides it. Not enthusiasm, not reassurance, but the actual mechanisms by which seated movement produces the same physiological changes that drive fat loss, improved energy, and better body composition in any other form of consistent practice.

The science is not complicated. The application is even simpler.

Why Most People Get This Wrong

The conventional model of exercise and weight loss is built around caloric burn. You move. You burn calories. If you burn more than you consume, you lose weight. This model is not wrong exactly, but it is incomplete in ways that matter particularly for older adults doing seated exercise.

Caloric burn during a seated Tai Chi session is modest. A ten-minute session will not produce the same acute caloric expenditure as a brisk walk or a cycling class. If caloric burn during the session were the only mechanism at work, the case for seated Tai Chi as a weight loss practice would be weak. But caloric burn during exercise is a minor fraction of the total energy story. The major levers are resting metabolic rate, hormonal environment, sleep quality, and what researchers call non-exercise activity thermogenesis, which is the energy your body uses for all movement that is not formal exercise.

Seated Tai Chi works through every one of these channels. It preserves and activates muscle tissue that keeps resting metabolic rate elevated. It lowers cortisol, which directly affects where and how the body stores fat. It improves sleep quality, which governs the hormonal environment that controls fat metabolism during the hours you are not practicing. And it typically increases overall movement and energy throughout the day, which raises NEAT in a way that accumulates meaningfully over time.

The resting metabolic rate explanation is worth sitting with for a moment. If sixty to seventy percent of daily calorie expenditure happens at rest, then the daily exercise session accounts for a much smaller portion of the body's total energy use than most people assume. A ten-minute seated session burns perhaps 25 to 40 calories during the session itself. But if that session activates muscle tissue that was previously dormant, raises resting metabolic rate for the following 24 hours, lowers cortisol for several hours, and improves sleep quality that night, the downstream effects on the body's total daily energy expenditure are considerably larger than the session's direct caloric cost. This is the framework within which seated Tai Chi makes physiological sense as a weight loss practice.

The mistake people make is evaluating any exercise practice solely by how hard it feels and how much they sweat. Intensity correlates with some benefits and actively undermines others. For an older adult whose cortisol is already elevated from poor sleep, chronic stress, and the accumulated demands of daily life, adding a high-intensity exercise session raises cortisol further, suppresses fat-burning hormones, and often disrupts sleep. The net effect can be an exercise practice that makes fat loss harder rather than easier. Seated Tai Chi does the opposite. It uses the body's own mechanisms to lower cortisol, improve hormonal balance, and create the conditions in which fat loss becomes progressively more possible.

This is not a consolation prize for people who cannot do harder things. It is the correct tool for the specific physiological situation that most people over sixty are in.

One more thing is worth saying plainly. High-intensity exercise for older adults often produces the cortisol problem it is trying to solve. A person who is already stressed, sleep-deprived, and carrying chronically elevated cortisol adds a significant cortisol spike every time they push through a hard workout. In younger adults the spike recovers in hours. In older adults it can persist well into the following day, suppressing fat-burning hormones and disrupting sleep. The person exercises harder, the cortisol stays high, and the weight does not move. Seated Tai Chi breaks this cycle rather than amplifying it.

What a Sedentary Body Actually Needs

Extended sitting, the kind that characterizes most sedentary daily life, produces specific physiological effects that accumulate over years. Understanding them is useful not as a source of concern but as a map of exactly what the practice is designed to address.

Reduced circulation.

When the large muscles of the legs are inactive for extended periods, the pumping action they provide to venous blood return slows. Blood pools in the lower extremities. The heart works harder to compensate. Lymphatic circulation, which depends almost entirely on muscle movement, slows and becomes less effective at clearing metabolic waste from the tissues. The result is a familiar cluster of symptoms: fatigue that is not explained by lack of sleep, swollen ankles, heaviness in the legs, and a general sense of reduced vitality that people often attribute to aging rather than to inactivity.

Seated Tai Chi addresses this directly. The deliberate movement of the arms, hips, and torso, combined with the rhythmic activation of the core and postural muscles, restores the pumping action that passive sitting removes. Even ten minutes of engaged seated movement measurably improves venous return and lymphatic circulation. This is one of the reasons many practitioners report feeling more alert and less fatigued within the first week of consistent practice.

Muscle deactivation.

Muscles that are not regularly engaged lose both mass and motor unit recruitment. The neural pathways that signal the muscles to activate become less efficient. This is the mechanism behind the functional weakness that many older adults experience: not disease, not injury, but simple disuse. The hip flexors shorten. The gluteal muscles become largely inactive during sitting. The deep core stabilizers that support the spine stop firing automatically. The result is poor sitting posture, lower back discomfort, and reduced stability when standing or walking.

The seated forms in Chapter Four are specifically designed to re-engage these systems. Each form activates the postural muscles, the hip rotators, and the deep core in a sequence that the nervous system begins to recognize and rebuild over repeated practice sessions. The strength that returns is functional: the kind that supports upright posture, makes rising from a chair easier, and reduces the energy cost of everyday movement.

Insulin resistance.

Prolonged physical inactivity reduces the muscles' sensitivity to insulin, the hormone that allows glucose to enter muscle cells for energy. When muscle cells are insulin-resistant, glucose stays in the bloodstream longer, drives higher insulin production, and is more likely to be converted to fat and stored. This is one of the metabolic pathways through which a sedentary lifestyle directly produces weight gain over time, independent of caloric intake.

Deliberate movement, even at low intensity, restores muscle insulin sensitivity in the hours following practice. Daily practice maintains this restored sensitivity consistently. The glucose that would otherwise circulate and be stored as fat gets used for the energy it was always intended to provide.

The important implication for older adults is that this mechanism operates independently of dietary change. You do not have to eat less to improve insulin sensitivity. You have to move more consistently. Ten minutes of deliberate seated movement, done every day, keeps the insulin sensitivity window open far more effectively than a 45-minute session done twice a week, because the daily practice never allows the muscle cells to fall back into the passive, insulin-resistant state that characterizes prolonged sedentary periods.

Elevated cortisol.

Passive sitting, particularly sitting associated with mental stress, financial worry, pain, or isolation, tends to maintain elevated cortisol levels. Chronically high cortisol drives abdominal fat storage, suppresses the hormones that support muscle preservation, and disrupts the sleep that the body uses to regulate its own hormonal environment. This is covered in detail in Chapter Two. The point here is that the problem is not movement alone. It is the hormonal environment that sedentary stress creates, and that seated Tai Chi addresses through its specific combination of deliberate movement and coordinated breathing.

Cortisol also affects appetite in specific ways. Chronically elevated cortisol increases cravings for high-calorie, high-carbohydrate foods, which are the foods that most directly contribute to the blood sugar spikes and insulin responses that drive fat storage. This is a biological mechanism, not a failure of willpower. When cortisol drops through consistent Tai Chi practice, these cravings often diminish without any deliberate dietary effort. People find themselves less drawn to the foods that were working against them, not because they restricted anything, but because the hormonal driver of those cravings has been reduced. This is one of the indirect ways the practice supports weight loss that most practitioners do not anticipate and do not attribute to the practice when it happens.

How Seated Movement Triggers Real Fat Loss

The mechanisms are straightforward. Each one is something you can feel when the practice is working.

Muscle activation raises resting metabolic rate.

The seated forms require sustained engagement of the postural muscles, the arms, the hips, and the core throughout each session. This is not intense effort. It is continuous low-level engagement. The muscles that are activated during practice burn additional calories at rest for hours afterward, because muscle tissue is metabolically expensive to maintain. Ten minutes of engaged seated movement does not produce dramatic acute caloric burn, but it does shift the resting metabolic rate in a direction that compounds over days and weeks of consistent practice.

Diaphragmatic breathing lowers cortisol.

Every form in Chapter Four is coordinated with diaphragmatic breathing. Deep abdominal breathing activates the vagus nerve, which in turn stimulates the parasympathetic nervous system. The parasympathetic state is the body's rest-and-digest mode: cortisol decreases, heart rate drops, digestion improves, and the hormonal conditions that drive fat storage shift toward those that support fat metabolism. This is not a subtle effect. Multiple peer-reviewed studies have measured cortisol reduction in older adults following Tai Chi practice. It is one of the most consistent findings in the research literature on this form of exercise.

Deliberate movement restores circulation.

Blood and lymphatic circulation improve during and after the forms. The improved circulation accelerates the clearance of inflammatory markers from the tissues, supports the delivery of nutrients to muscle cells, and produces the subjective experience of warmth and lightness that many practitioners describe after a session. Better circulation also supports fat metabolism by improving the delivery of oxygen to tissues where fat oxidation occurs.

Core engagement improves posture and energy efficiency.

The seated forms are anchored in a specific postural foundation: spine lengthened, core gently engaged, shoulders back and down. This posture is itself a form of strength training for the deep stabilizers of the back and abdomen. People who maintain this posture through a session use more muscular effort than they realize, and the carryover into the rest of the day, when they sit more easily and with less spinal load, reduces fatigue and increases the energy available for other activity.

Over several weeks of consistent practice, many people find that they sit better outside of the practice as well. The upright posture begins to feel natural rather than forced. The days of slouching into a chair without noticing it become less frequent. This is a postural change, but it is also an energy change: a body that is not fighting against its own collapsed posture has more resources available for everything else.

The Independence Factor

There is a dimension to this practice that the physiology cannot fully capture, and it deserves a direct word.

For many people reading this book, the ability to exercise independently, without needing equipment, a gym, a trainer, or another person's help, has become uncertain. Joint problems, balance conditions, post-surgical recovery, or simply the accumulated physical caution that comes with age have made the forms of exercise that were once available feel risky or inaccessible. That loss is real. It is not trivial, and it is not imagined.

What seated Tai Chi offers, practically, is a path back to independent movement. Not a consolation version of exercise. Not something to do until something better becomes possible. A complete practice that produces documented health benefits and that can be done alone, in any room, without help from anyone, for as long as the practitioner chooses to continue.

I have watched people who came to a seated practice because they had no other options decide, over time, that it was the option they would have chosen anyway. The practice asks for attention more than for physical capacity. It rewards consistency more than intensity. It is well-suited to the patient and deliberate engagement that older adults bring to almost everything they do. These are not compensations for limitations. They are genuine advantages.

The chair practice in this book is not a lesser version of standing Tai Chi. It is a version developed specifically for the seated body, with forms chosen and adapted to produce the full range of benefits from that position. The research on seated Tai Chi in older adults supports this directly: participants in seated programs show measurable improvements in muscle strength, flexibility, balance (even when assessed only while seated), cortisol levels, sleep quality, and self-reported energy. The practice is complete in itself.

The research on seated Tai Chi in older adults supports this directly. Studies in clinical settings have documented significant improvements in muscle strength, range of motion, cortisol levels, sleep quality, and self-reported energy and mood in participants who practiced seated Tai Chi consistently for as few as four weeks. The results in home practice settings are comparable, which means the benefit is not dependent on clinical supervision or a specially equipped environment. A chair in a living room is sufficient.

Independence is not just a practical matter. For many older adults, the capacity to care for their own bodies without assistance is one of the most important remaining dimensions of autonomy. Maintaining it, or recovering some portion of it after a period of decline, has psychological and emotional weight that physical measurements cannot fully capture. This practice offers a genuine path toward that maintenance, and it does so in a way that can be continued indefinitely, without equipment wearing out, without gym memberships lapsing, and without the need for anyone else's schedule or assistance.

There is also something worth naming about the relationship between physical agency and psychological wellbeing. People who cannot move their bodies independently tend to internalize that limitation in ways that extend beyond the physical. The willingness to try new things narrows. Social confidence often decreases. The sense of being a person who takes care of themselves, which most older adults held for decades, becomes uncertain. When movement becomes possible again, even modest deliberate seated movement, these psychological effects reverse in ways that are disproportionate to the physical change. People describe feeling like themselves again. That phrase carries a lot.

Whatever brought you to this book, the practice it contains is worth your ten minutes. Not because ten minutes is all your body is worth, but because ten consistent daily minutes will produce more change over 28 days than any ambitious program that gets abandoned on Day 6. The chair is the starting point. The practice is what it leads to. And the practice, it turns out, belongs to anyone willing to sit in a chair and begin.

Chapter 2

What's Happening Inside Your Body

The forms in Chapter Four work whether or not you understand why they work. But knowing why tends to keep people practicing, especially on the days when the motivation is low and the reason matters.

This chapter explains the physiology in plain terms. No clinical distance. No promises. Just what is actually happening when a person who has been sedentary begins ten minutes of consistent deliberate seated movement every day.

Your Metabolism at Rest and How to Wake It Up

Metabolism is not a single thing. It is a collection of processes, and resting metabolic rate, the calories the body burns simply to stay alive, is by far the largest component. For most people, resting metabolic rate accounts for sixty to seventy percent of total daily calorie expenditure. Exercise, even significant exercise, accounts for a much smaller portion. This means that the most powerful way to shift the body's total energy expenditure is not to exercise harder. It is to shift the resting metabolic rate.

Muscle is the primary driver of resting metabolic rate. Every pound of muscle the body maintains burns approximately six calories per day at rest. Fat tissue burns roughly two. As muscle mass decreases with age and inactivity, resting metabolic rate falls. The body burns fewer calories at rest. The same food intake that maintained weight at fifty produces weight gain at sixty-five, not because eating changed but because the body's composition did.

Seated Tai Chi addresses this directly. The sustained low-load engagement of the postural muscles, the arm muscles, the hip rotators, and the deep core throughout every session stimulates the nervous system's signals to maintain and gradually rebuild these muscle groups. This is not the dramatic muscle gain produced by heavy resistance training. It is the kind of steady functional muscle preservation that keeps the metabolism running at a sustainable rate and that makes daily movement feel less effortful over time.

NEAT responds to the practice in ways that are easy to overlook. A person who finishes a ten-minute seated session feeling more alert and less fatigued than when they started tends to do more throughout the rest of the day. They get up to refill their glass instead of waiting. They shift position more often. They are more willing to walk to another room rather than letting something wait. Each of these movements is small. Accumulated across an entire day, they represent a meaningful additional energy expenditure that the formal session itself does not account for.

Non-exercise activity thermogenesis, the energy used for all daily movement that is not formal exercise, also responds to the practice. People who feel more energetic after a consistent movement practice tend to move more throughout the day without thinking about it. They stand up more readily. They walk across the room instead of waiting. They fidget less from discomfort and more from a body that is ready to move. These accumulated micro-movements add up to a meaningful additional calorie expenditure that the session itself does not fully account for. The practice changes the resting baseline, and the resting baseline drives the majority of the body's daily energy equation.

Breath, Cortisol, and Where Fat Actually Goes

This is the most important mechanism in the book, and it is worth reading carefully.

Cortisol is the body's primary stress hormone. Its job is to mobilize energy rapidly in response to a perceived threat. It raises blood sugar, suppresses digestion, accelerates heart rate, and puts the body on high alert. In short bursts, this is useful. The problem is chronic elevation.

For a significant number of older adults, particularly those managing chronic pain, social isolation, financial stress, disrupted sleep, or the accumulated weight of caregiving or loss, cortisol is not spiking and recovering. It is elevated as a baseline state, persisting at levels that were designed to be temporary but have become continuous. Chronic cortisol elevation produces a specific cluster of effects: abdominal fat accumulation, suppression of the hormones that support muscle preservation, disrupted sleep, elevated inflammatory markers, and reduced insulin sensitivity.

The abdominal fat connection is particularly direct. Cortisol activates receptors in the deep abdominal fat tissue that stimulate fat storage in that area. This is the mechanism behind the visceral fat accumulation that tends to accelerate after sixty, and it is why people whose diet and exercise have not dramatically changed sometimes find that their body composition shifts noticeably in their mid-sixties. It is hormonal, not merely caloric.

Diaphragmatic breathing is one of the most effective cortisol interventions available. When the diaphragm expands fully on the inhale, it activates stretch receptors that send signals through the vagus nerve to the brainstem. The brainstem responds by activating the parasympathetic nervous system. Heart rate slows. Blood pressure drops. Cortisol production decreases. The body shifts out of the stress state and into a state where repair, digestion, and fat metabolism are prioritized over storage and defense.

The breathing in Chapter Three teaches this exactly. Every seated form in Chapter Four is coordinated with diaphragmatic breath. Ten minutes of practice involves dozens of full diaphragmatic breath cycles. The cortisol reduction from a single session is measurable and lasts for several hours. Daily practice begins to shift the resting cortisol baseline over weeks. The abdominal fat that cortisol was driving begins to respond to that shifted baseline. This is the central fat loss mechanism in this practice, and it requires nothing from the practitioner except the willingness to breathe deliberately for ten minutes.

Why Seated Bodies Struggle With Circulation and Energy

Prolonged sitting compresses the large blood vessels of the thighs and restricts venous return from the lower extremities. The calf muscles, which normally act as a secondary pump helping push blood back toward the heart, are inactive. The lymphatic system, which has no pump of its own and depends entirely on muscle movement to circulate fluid, slows dramatically. The result is that metabolic waste products accumulate in the tissues of the legs and lower back, producing the familiar fatigue, heaviness, and stiffness that many older adults experience by mid-morning after sitting since they woke.

Synovial fluid, the lubricant that keeps joints moving without friction, is produced in response to joint movement. Joints that are held in one position for extended periods produce less fluid. The stiffness people experience after sitting for an hour is not just muscular. It is partly the joints losing their lubrication from the absence of movement. The first movements after a long sit feel stiff because they are partly the joints re-generating the fluid they need.

The seated forms address all of these systems simultaneously. The movement of the arms activates the postural muscles of the upper back and core, which improves thoracic circulation. The hip circles and waist turns engage the hip flexors and rotators, restoring blood flow to the compressed structures of the pelvis and thighs. The ankle and knee movements in the Circulation Builders section of Chapter Four directly activate the calf pump mechanism and promote lymphatic drainage from the lower legs.

The Circulation Builders in Chapter Four, three short movements specifically designed to address venous return and lymphatic drainage, are placed at the end of the form sequence for this reason. After the main forms have activated the postural and core muscles, the Circulation Builders direct specific attention to the ankle joints, the knee flexors, and the shoulder girdle. These are the structures most compressed and least activated during ordinary sitting. Five minutes of deliberate attention to them at the end of each session changes how the legs feel for the rest of the day.

Postural muscle engagement also has a cumulative structural benefit. As the deep stabilizers of the spine and hips strengthen through consistent seated practice, the body holds itself more upright automatically. Better posture reduces the compressive load on the lumbar spine, which in turn reduces the chronic low-level pain that many older adults carry and that contributes to the hormonal stress load keeping cortisol elevated. The improvement in posture is both a result of the practice and a mechanism by which the practice continues to improve the hormonal environment.

Ten minutes of this kind of engaged movement, done daily, changes the baseline. The stiffness that took until noon to resolve begins resolving by nine. The afternoon energy drop becomes less pronounced. The heaviness in the legs at the end of the day reduces. These are circulation and lymphatic effects, and they arrive before any significant change in body composition does. They are the first evidence that the practice is working.

What 28 Days of Consistent Gentle Movement Does

The timeline of adaptation to a new movement practice follows a recognizable pattern. Understanding it prevents the disappointment of expecting the wrong things at the wrong time.

Week One: the nervous system responds.

The first week of any new movement practice produces primarily neural adaptations. The nervous system learns the patterns of the forms, begins firing the appropriate motor units in the appropriate sequence, and starts establishing the habit signal that brings you back to the chair the following morning. Sleep often improves in the first week, because the cortisol reduction from even a few sessions of diaphragmatic breathing practice begins shifting the nighttime hormonal environment. Most people notice something by Day 3 or 4, usually in the quality of a morning or the speed at which the body warms up.

Weeks Two and Three: the muscles respond.

By the second and third weeks, the motor patterns are more established and the postural muscles begin sustaining their activation more efficiently. The seated forms feel less effortful to coordinate. The body holds the upright posture more naturally. The hip muscles, which may have been largely inactive for years, begin contributing to the movements in ways that produce a genuine sense of engagement. Cortisol reduction effects are now consistent rather than intermittent. Many people notice changes in appetite regulation, since lower cortisol reduces the hormonal drive toward high-calorie comfort foods that accompanies chronic stress.

Week Four: body composition begins to shift.

By the fourth week, the combination of improved muscle activation, consistently lower cortisol, better sleep, and improved insulin sensitivity creates the conditions in which body composition genuinely begins to change. This does not always show up on the scale. Muscle gained offsets fat lost on a scale. But it shows up in how clothing fits, in how the body moves, and in the energy available for the rest of the day. Some people see the scale move. Some see it stay the same while their body is noticeably different. Both are real progress.

The most honest thing that can be said about what 28 days produces is this: it establishes the conditions for continued improvement. The cortisol baseline is lower. The muscle activation patterns are re-established. The sleep is better. The insulin sensitivity is improved. The nervous system has the movement patterns in place. None of these gains require the program to continue in its original structured form. They require the practice to continue, in whatever adapted form suits the practitioner's life. A ten-minute daily session is enough to sustain and build on all of the physiological changes produced in the first 28 days.

Chapter Eight addresses what comes after Day 28 in detail. For now, what matters is the understanding that the 28 days are not the destination. They are the foundation. The practice built in 28 days can be maintained for years and improved across decades. The chair will always be there. The forms are yours as long as you practice them.

Be honest with yourself about the timeline. Twenty-eight days of consistent practice produces real and measurable change. It does not produce dramatic transformation. The purpose of 28 days is to establish a practice that continues past Day 28, and the cumulative effects of three months, six months, and a year of consistent seated Tai Chi are what produces the changes most people are hoping for when they start. The program gets you to the starting line. What you do with the practice after Day 28 is where the real change accumulates.

Chapter 3

Setting Up for Success

Before the first form, before the first breath of deliberate practice, there are a few things worth getting right. They take ten minutes to sort out once, and they make every session after that more comfortable and more effective.

Your Chair, Your Space, Your Starting Line

The chair is not incidental. It is the foundation of everything in this program, and the wrong chair will undermine the practice before it begins.

The right chair.

Choose a chair with no arms. Arms interfere with the sweeping movements of several forms and prevent the full range of shoulder and hip rotation the practice requires. The seat must be firm, not cushioned deeply enough that the pelvis sinks into it. When the pelvis is unsupported and unlevel, the spine cannot lengthen correctly, and the postural engagement that makes the seated forms effective is compromised from the start.

Seat height matters. When seated, your feet should rest flat on the floor with your knees at approximately a right angle, not angled sharply upward as they would be in a chair that is too low, and not dangling as they would in one that is too high. A standard dining chair works for most people. If the seat is slightly too high, a thin non-slip mat under the feet resolves it. If it is too low, a firm cushion on the seat brings the height up.

The chair must not move during practice. If it slides on a hard floor, place a non-slip mat underneath it or practice on carpet. Stability is not a preference. It is a safety requirement.

Your space.

Position the chair in a clear area with enough room to extend both arms fully forward and to each side without touching anything. You need at least two feet of clearance on each side and three feet in front. You do not need a large room. A corner of a bedroom, a cleared kitchen area, or any open living space works. The floor under the chair should be level.

If possible, practice in a space with some natural light. This is not essential. What is essential is that the space feels calm enough to sustain ten minutes of attention. Some people practice near a window. Some face a plain wall. The practice itself creates the environment once it begins.

Keep the chair in the same place. This is a small thing that has a larger effect than it seems. When the chair is always in the same spot, the decision to practice is already half made before you sit down. The consistency of place supports the consistency of habit.

> **Jing's Note**
> Getting the chair right is not fussy preparation. It is the same principle as getting the forms right: precision in the setup makes everything that follows more effective. Spend five minutes on this once. Then forget about the chair and pay attention to the practice.

Sitting Tall

The most important skill in this entire program is not a form. It is a sitting position. Every form in Chapter Four begins and ends here. Getting it into the body before Day 1 is the best preparation you can do.

The position is called the Tai Chi seated neutral. It is not ramrod-straight posture. It is not relaxed slouching. It is a specific, sustainable alignment that lets the spine do its job without effort.

Starting Position:

Sit toward the front half of your chair. Your hips should be near the front edge of the seat, not pushed back against the chair back. Both feet flat on the floor, hip-width apart, toes pointing forward or slightly outward. Hands resting on thighs.

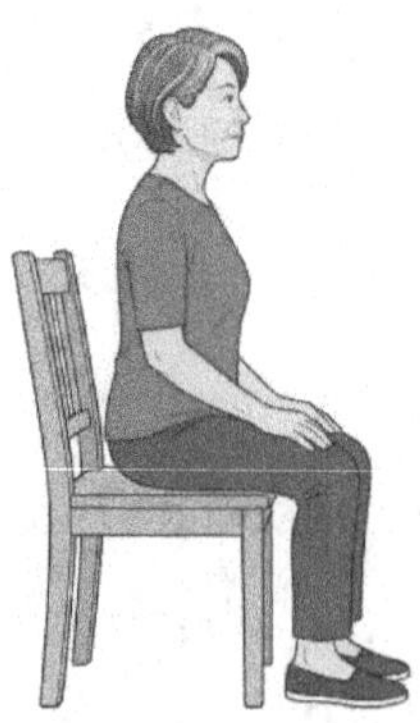

Steps:

1. Press both feet evenly into the floor. Feel the floor beneath the heel, the ball of the foot, and all five toes without gripping.

2. Gently tilt the pelvis slightly forward, finding the natural curve of the lower back. Not an exaggerated arch, not a flat plank. A comfortable, natural curve.

3. Allow the spine to lengthen upward from that base. Imagine a thread attached to the crown of your head, drawing you lightly upward.

4. Let the shoulders drop away from the ears. Roll them back slightly so the chest opens. The shoulder blades settle toward each other without squeezing.

5. Bring the chin to a level position, parallel to the floor. The gaze rests forward at eye height, soft and unfocused.

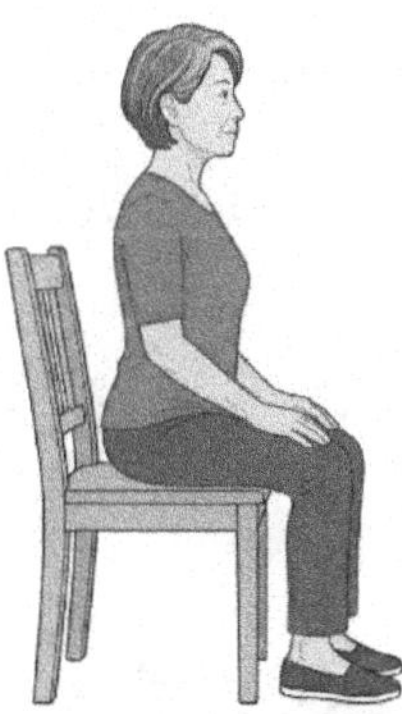

6. Hold this position and take three slow breaths. Notice where you feel the postural muscles engaging. The lower back, the deep core, the muscles between the shoulder blades. These are the muscles the practice is building.

BREATHING: Breathe naturally throughout. The posture should feel sustainable, not effortful.

FEEL IT: A mild engagement in the deep back and core muscles. A slight lift across the chest. The neck long and free rather than compressed.

IF NEEDED: If maintaining the front-of-seat position is difficult, sit further back toward the middle of the seat and focus on the spinal lengthening without worrying about the pelvis position. Approach the full neutral gradually over the first few days.

Breathing as a Weight Loss Tool

The breath is not background noise in this practice. It is the mechanism by which the cortisol reduction described in Chapter Two actually happens. Learning diaphragmatic breathing before Day 1 means the practice works from the very first session rather than after several sessions of getting used to the coordination.

Diaphragmatic breathing is the natural breath of the relaxed body. Most adults breathe primarily into the chest: the shoulders rise, the upper ribs expand, and the belly stays still or even draws in. This pattern is efficient for stress states, when the body is ready for action. It is not efficient for recovery, metabolism regulation, or cortisol clearance. Belly breathing, in which the diaphragm descends on the inhale and the abdomen expands, signals the nervous system that the threat has passed and the parasympathetic state can activate.

Starting Position:

Seated in Tai Chi neutral. One hand placed flat on the lower abdomen just below the navel, the other hand resting on the thigh.

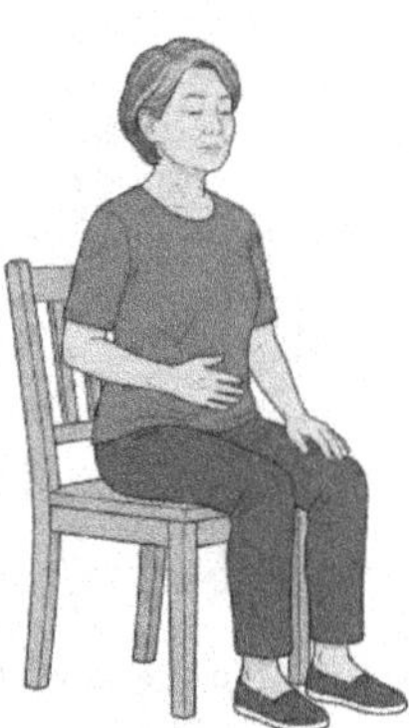

Steps:

1. Start with an exhale. Open the lips slightly and let the air go out completely. The belly eases inward on its own as the air exits.

2. Start the inhale through the nose. The breath should be directed downward, not upward. The hand resting on the abdomen should push outward as the belly rises. The chest barely moves, just slightly.

3. Take four slow counts to complete the inhale. The belly leads, then the lower ribs open, then the chest rises last.

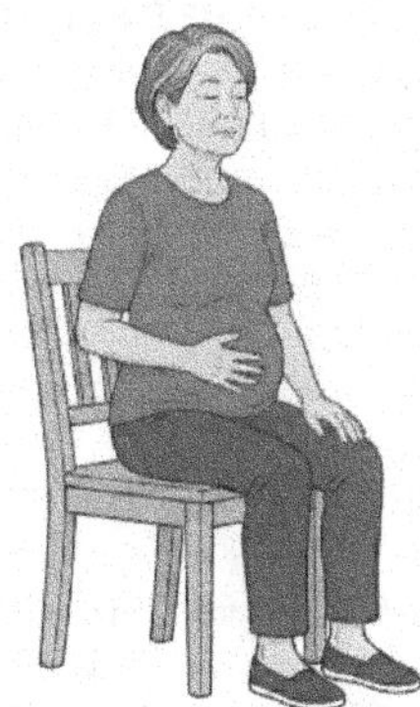

4. Hold quietly at the top for one count. No forcing, just a brief, natural pause.

5. Exhale through slightly parted lips for six counts. The belly pulls back in. The ribs settle. The shoulders remain still and level.

6. Pause at the bottom for one count before the next inhale begins.

7. Repeat for six complete cycles. When done with the sixth exhale, let the breath revert to its natural rhythm.

BREATHING: This exercise IS the breathing practice. Inhale four counts, exhale six. The longer exhale is where the parasympathetic activation occurs.

FEEL IT: A quieting sensation beginning around the third or fourth cycle. Some people notice a slight warmth across the chest. The hand on the belly moves noticeably outward on the inhale and falls back on the exhale.

IF NEEDED: Let go of the counting entirely if it is getting in the way. What matters is the direction: breathe into the belly, and exhale longer than you inhale. This is more important than the actual count.

Jing's Note

This breathing practice can be used any time, not only during sessions. Two minutes of this breath before a difficult situation, before sleep, or during a stressful afternoon produces measurable cortisol reduction. The forms make it more systematic. But the breath alone is a tool you can use anywhere.

Pain, Stiffness, and Difficult Days

Any 28-day program will include days when the body is less cooperative than usual. Knowing in advance what to do on those days removes the decision from the morning, when motivation and flexibility are at their lowest.

General morning stiffness.

Waking up stiff is a normal part of mornings for most people over sixty, and it tells you very little about how the rest of the day will feel. The joints need a few minutes of movement before the lubricating fluid inside them redistributes properly. If you practice first thing, simply start with the Sitting Tall exercise and the breathing practice slowly than you normally would; smaller movements, softer effort and give the body a few minutes to warm into the session. By the time the breathing practice is complete, the stiffness will have largely resolved on its own. Do not skip the session because of morning stiffness. The practice is the remedy, not the obstacle.

Joint-specific pain.

If a specific joint is painful on a given day, use the IF NEEDED modification for any form that engages that joint. For shoulder pain, reduce the range of arm movements. For hip pain, reduce the depth of the hip circles and waist turns. For lower back discomfort, focus particularly on the Sitting Tall alignment before beginning and check it again mid-session. Sharp pain that does not ease within a minute of modifying the movement is the signal to stop that movement, not to push through it.

Low-energy days.

On days when energy is genuinely low, the session changes but does not disappear. Do the Sitting Tall exercise, the breathing practice, and the Seated Closing Form only. That is three minutes. The cortisol reduction from the breathing practice alone is worth the three minutes, and the habit of showing up regardless of energy is one of the things that keeps a practice alive past Day 28.

Where You Are Right Now

Before Day 1, take five minutes to do this assessment. Write the results down. These four measures are the baselines for the progress checks in Chapter Five. They are not tests with passing grades. They are starting points.

Measure 1 – Seated Reach

Sit in Tai Chi neutral. Raise both arms forward to shoulder height, palms facing each other. Without leaning, reach forward slowly until you feel a stretch in the backs of the arms or across the shoulders. Note roughly how far your fingertips extend past your knees: level with the knees, a hand's width past, further.

1. Sit in Tai Chi neutral, feet flat, spine long.

2. Raise both arms to shoulder height, palms facing each other.

3. Reach forward slowly without rounding the spine. Hold where you feel a first stretch.

4. Note the result. Return to neutral.

Measure 2 – Hip Rotation Range

Still seated, place both hands on your thighs. Slowly rotate your upper body to the right as far as is comfortable, keeping the hips stable. Note how far you can turn: shoulders past the knee, to the knee, only partway. Repeat left.

1. Hands on thighs, feet flat, spine long.

2. Turn the upper body slowly to the right. Hips stay facing forward.

3. Note the point where rotation stops comfortably. Return to center.

4. Repeat to the left. Note the comparison.

Measure 3 – Breath Hold Comfortable Pause

After a full diaphragmatic inhale, pause at the top of the breath. Count how many seconds you can hold comfortably before the inhale urge becomes strong. This is not a breath-hold challenge. It is a measure of baseline breath capacity.

1. Take one full diaphragmatic inhale as practiced earlier.

2. Pause at the top naturally, without forcing.

3. Count quietly until the urge to exhale becomes noticeable.

4. Note the count. A comfortable pause of 3 to 5 seconds is typical. More or less are both normal starting points.

Measure 4 – Energy Self-Rating

On a scale of 1 to 5, how would you rate your typical morning energy over the past week? One means very low, barely functional. Five means clear and ready. Write the number. You will answer this same question at Days 13, 20, and 28.

Important

These four baselines are the benchmarks for the Chapter Five progress checks. Write them somewhere you can find them. If you do not write them down, the progress checks at Days 13, 20, and 28 will have nothing to measure against.

Chapter 4

The Seated Forms

Think of this chapter as your reference shelf. Every seated form used in the 28-day program lives here, written out completely, step by step, so you always have somewhere to turn when the program calls for a movement you want to review. Before Day 1, read through it once from start to finish. Not to memorize, just to familiarize. When you meet a form in the program, it will already feel like something you have seen before.

How to Read the Instructions

Every form in this chapter follows the same layout. The starting position is described in prose first. The first image appears immediately after that description and shows you what the position looks like before the steps begin. Then the numbered steps follow. Additional images appear within the steps at the specific moment they correspond to, so you can read a step, look at the image, and see the position being described.

Each set of instructions closes with three short cues. BREATHING lays out when to draw breath in and when to release it during the movement. FEEL IT gives you a physical checkpoint — what the movement should register as in the body when it is being done well. IF NEEDED offers a scaled-down version for days when the body needs more room.

Every form assumes you are seated. There are no standing versions in this chapter. The forms are complete as seated exercises and are designed to produce their full benefits from the chair.

After the eight forms, you will find the Core and Posture Engagement section, which explains the muscle engagement that underlies the practice, and the Circulation Builders section, three short movements specifically designed to address circulation and lymphatic drainage from the seated position. All three Circulation Builders together take less than five minutes and are worth reading before Week Three, when they first appear in the program.

The Eight Core Seated Forms

Form 1 – Seated Cloud Hands

The foundational weight-shift form. Trains the lateral transfer of weight through the pelvis and hips while coordinating continuous arm movement. This is the form that ties the practice together and appears in every week of the program.

Starting Position:

Sit in Tai Chi neutral. Both hands rest at your sides at hip level, palms facing slightly inward. Your weight is evenly distributed across both sit bones.

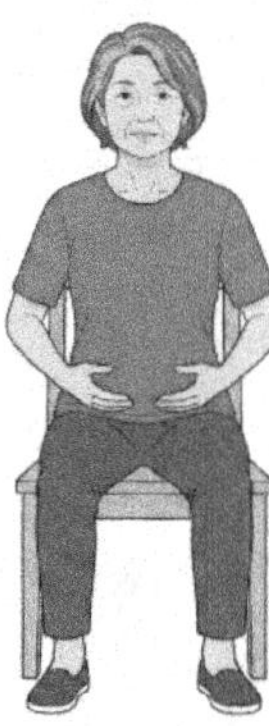

Steps:

1. Raise your right hand in a slow arc to chest height, palm facing inward toward the body. Simultaneously let the left hand rest at hip height, palm facing gently downward.

2. Begin shifting your weight slightly onto the right sit bone as the right hand continues its arc across the front of the body toward the left.

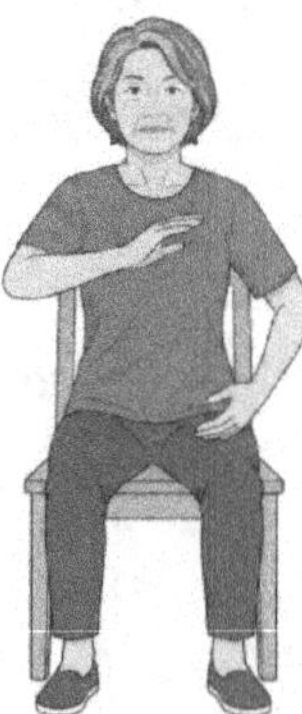

3. As the right hand reaches the left side and begins to descend, raise the left hand to chest height and begin shifting weight back toward the left sit bone.

4. The left hand sweeps across to the right at chest height as the right hand descends to hip level. Weight shifts with the arc.

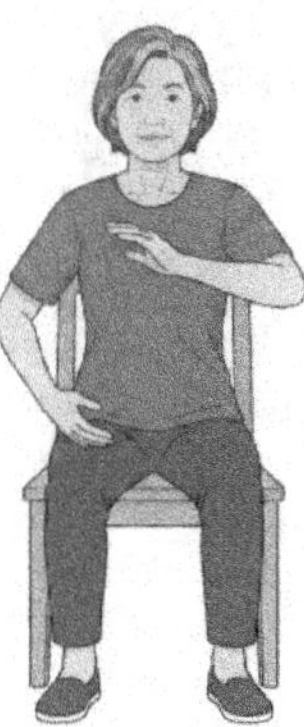

5. Continue this alternating sweep for eight full cycles. Neither hand stops. The movement flows continuously, each arc completing into the next.

6. After the eighth cycle, settle both hands at hip level and hold for one breath.

BREATHING: Inhale as each hand rises. Exhale as it sweeps across and descends. One full breath per side.

FEEL IT: A gentle warmth developing through the hips and lower back as the weight shifts. The arms float rather than being lifted. The waist follows the arc of the arms.

IF NEEDED: Reduce the range of the weight shift if hip pain is present. The arm arc can be performed without any lateral weight transfer and still produces the upper-body benefit.

Complete eight cycles.

Form 2 – Dragon Stirs the Waters

A slow continuous hip circle that lubricates the hip joints, activates the deep hip rotators, and restores synovial fluid to the pelvis and lower back.

Starting Position:

Sit in Tai Chi neutral, feet flat and hip-width apart. Both hands rest on the tops of the thighs near the knees.

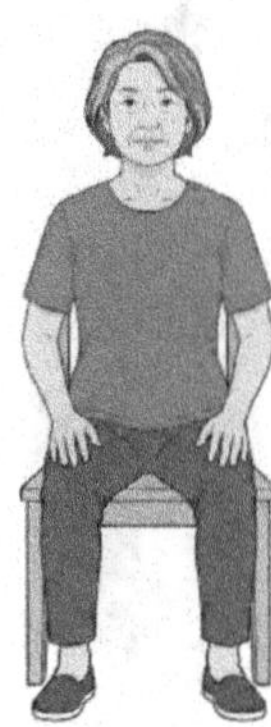

Steps:

1. Begin a slow horizontal circle with the pelvis, as though tracing a circle on the seat of the chair with your sit bones. Start by shifting the pelvis slightly forward.

2. Continue the circle to the right, shifting the weight toward the right sit bone. The movement comes from the hips, not the shoulders.

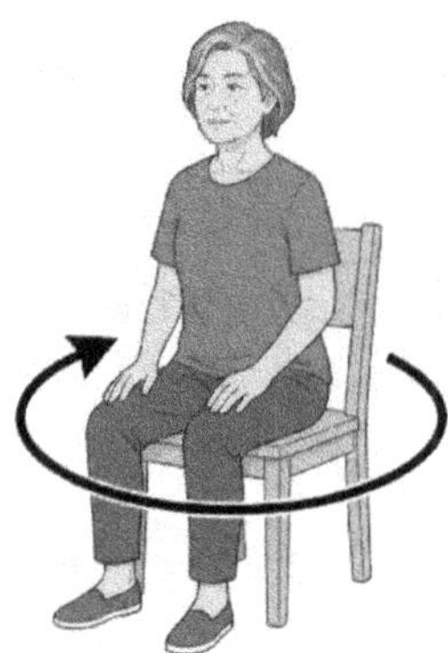

3. Continue the arc rearward, shifting the pelvis slightly backward and to the left.

4. Complete the circle back to center and continue into the next rotation.

5. Complete five full circles in one direction. Slow and deliberate, not rushed.

6. Pause at center for one breath.

7. Reverse direction for five more circles.

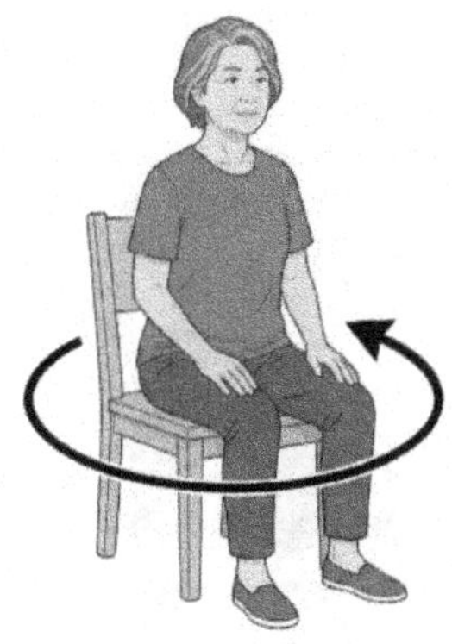

BREATHING: No specific pattern needed here. Keep the breathing normally. If you find yourself holding it at any point, exhale completely and let the next inhale arrive on its own.

FEEL IT: A loosening warmth through the hip joints and lower back. Some people feel a mild release in the sacroiliac area. This is normal and is the effect of the joint receiving movement it rarely gets.

IF NEEDED: Reduce the diameter of the circle if any point in the rotation produces sharp discomfort. Even a small circle lubricates the joint.

Five circles each direction.

Form 3 – Lotus Arms

Opens the chest and shoulder girdle, improves thoracic circulation, and trains the slow coordinated arm extension that runs through several of the more complex forms.

Starting Position:

Sit in Tai Chi neutral. Both hands gathered loosely in the lap, right hand over left, palms facing upward.

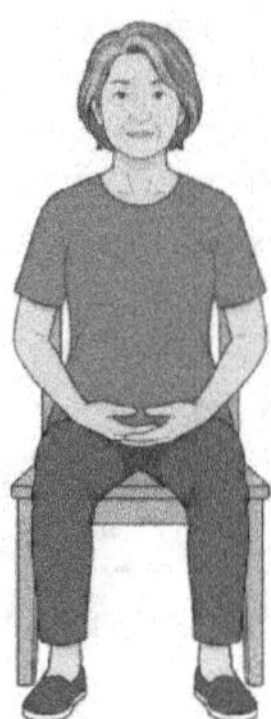

Steps:

1. On a slow inhale, begin raising both arms outward from the sides, like wings opening. Palms face upward as the arms rise.

2. Continue raising until both arms reach shoulder height, extended out to each side. Pause.

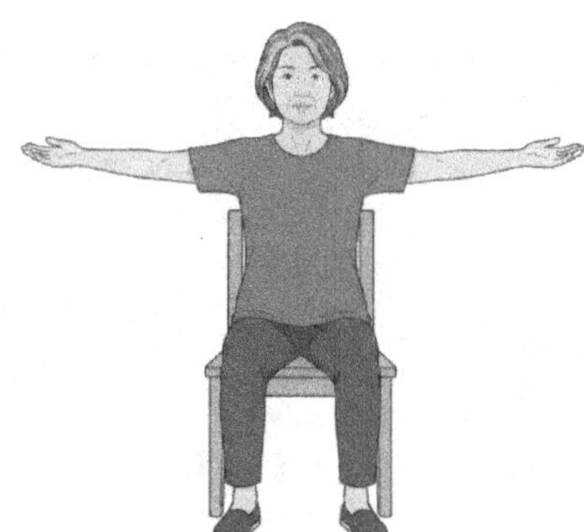

3. Flip the palms to face the downward and begin the descent on the exhale, pressing downward steadily as though the air itself has some resistance to it.

4. When the arms return to hip level, begin rotating the palms to face inward and bring both hands together in front of the lower abdomen in a gathering motion.

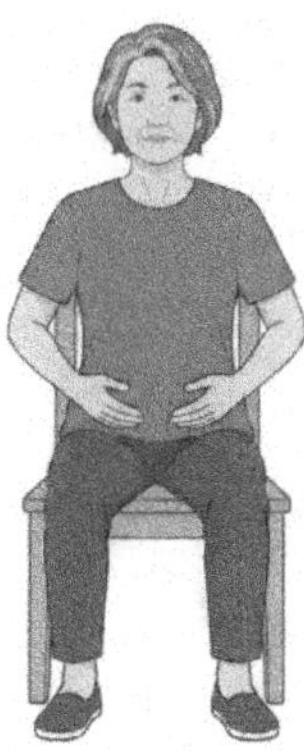

5. Pause for one breath with hands gathered at the abdomen.

6. Repeat the full cycle. Complete six repetitions.

BREATHING: Inhale as the arms open and rise. Exhale as they press down and gather.

FEEL IT: A clear opening across the chest and front of the shoulders on the rise. A gentle pressing sensation as the arms lower. Some people feel a warmth in the hands from the increased circulation.

IF NEEDED: Reduce the height of the arm rise if shoulder pain is present. Arms raised to 45 degrees rather than full shoulder height produces the same chest-opening benefit with less shoulder load.

Complete six repetitions.

Form 4 – Seated Single Whip

A lateral extension form that trains the postural muscles of the upper back, opens the chest across a wide range, and builds sustained arm strength through held positions.

Starting Position:

Sit in Tai Chi neutral. Gather the fingers of the right hand together into a loose downward-pointing beak shape, fingertips touching, wrist relaxed. Extend this arm to the right at shoulder height. The left arm rests at the left side.

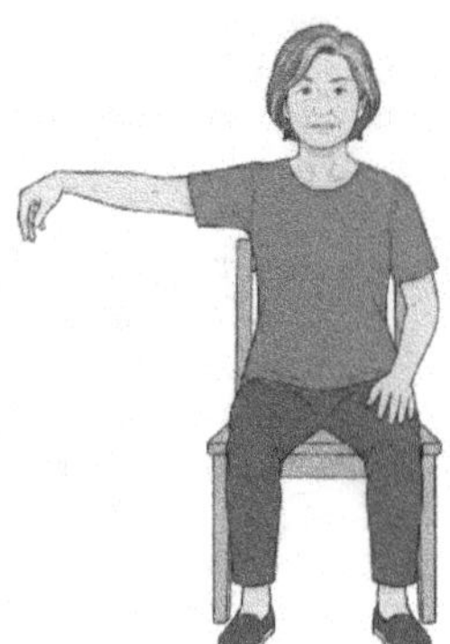

Steps:

1. Raise the left arm forward to shoulder height, palm facing to the right. Simultaneously turn the head gently to look toward the left hand.

2. Hold this extended position for two full breaths. Right arm extended to the right in beak position. Left arm extended forward. Chest wide and open.

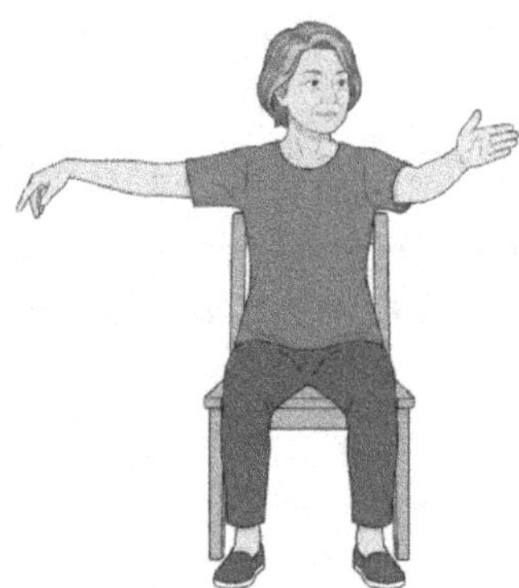

3. Lower both arms and settle for one breath.

4. Set up the left-side repetition: left arm extended to the left in beak position, right arm raised forward, head turned right.

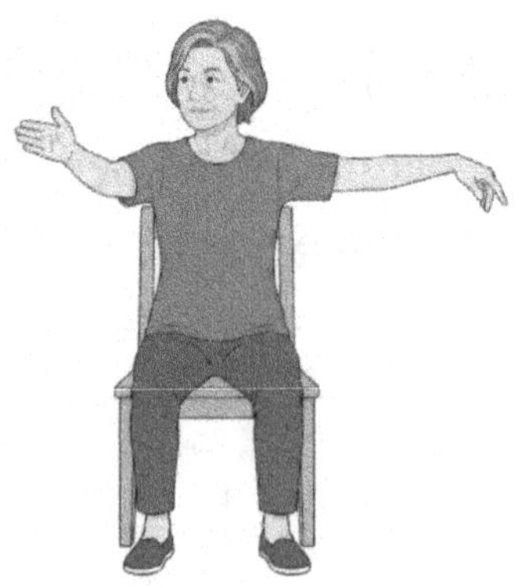

5. Hold for two full breaths.

6. Complete three repetitions each side.

BREATHING: Inhale as you extend. Hold naturally at the extended position. Exhale as you lower.

FEEL IT: A clear engagement across the upper back between the shoulder blades. The chest opens between the two extended arms. A steady engagement in the extended arms after the first breath.

IF NEEDED: Reduce the hold to one breath if two feels like too much for the shoulder girdle. Build to two breaths over the first two weeks.

Three repetitions each side.

Form 5 – Gathering the Sky

A full upward reach form that decompresses the spine, opens the ribcage for fuller diaphragmatic breathing, and trains the lengthening posture that the seated practice builds toward.

Starting Position:

Sit in Tai Chi neutral. Both hands rest in the lap, palms upward.

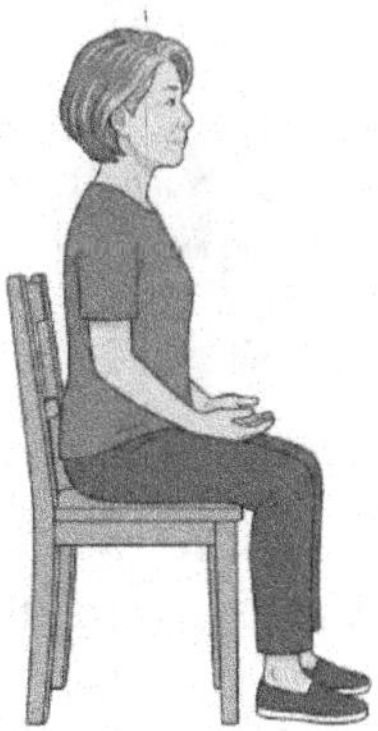

Steps:

1. On a slow inhale, bring both hands together at the lower abdomen and begin raising them upward along the centerline of the body, palms facing upward as if lifting something gently.

2. Continue raising until both arms are fully extended overhead, palms facing each other. At full height, pause and feel the spine lengthen.

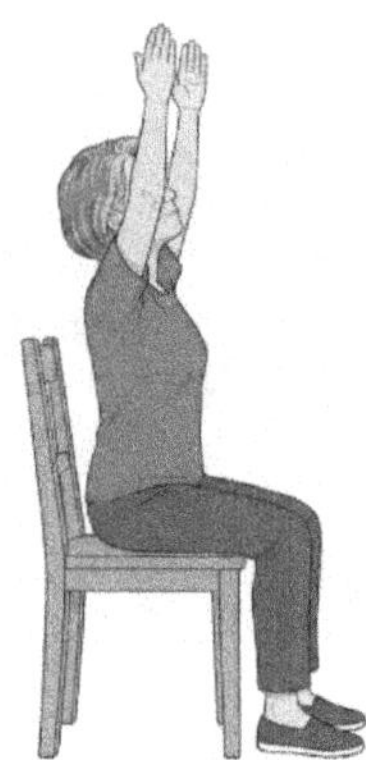

3. Turn the palms outward to face away from each other.

4. On a slow exhale, open both arms outward and downward in a wide arc, like wings descending, pressing down through the air.

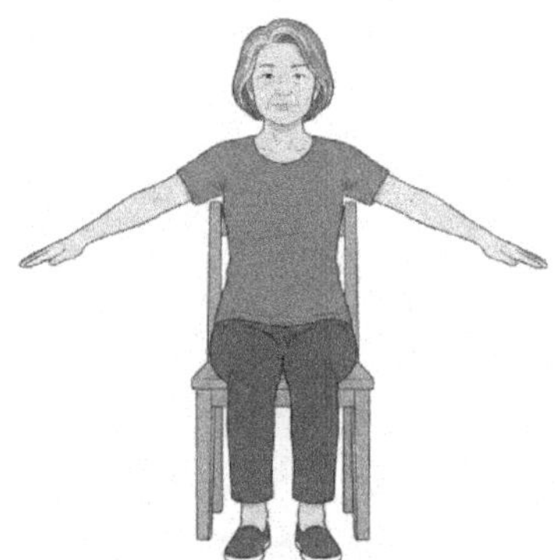

5. As the hands return to lap level, turn the palms upward to receive the next rise.

6. Complete six repetitions. Slow and continuous, breath driving every movement.

BREATHING: Inhale on the rise. Exhale on the descent. Let the breath guide the pace of the movement rather than the movement guiding the breath.

FEEL IT: A clear decompression in the lower back and thoracic spine at full reach. Many people feel the ribcage expand noticeably on the full inhale at the top. This is the diaphragm accessing its full range.

IF NEEDED: Reduce the overhead extension if shoulder or neck discomfort prevents a full reach. Arms raised to forehead height rather than fully overhead produces most of the spinal decompression benefit.

Six repetitions.

Form 6 – Hip Circle Flow

An extended hip rotation sequence that combines the Dragon Stirs the Waters circle with an arm coordination layer, building the simultaneous hip and arm movement that characterizes more advanced Tai Chi work.

Starting Position:

Sit in Tai Chi neutral. Left hand rests at hip level, right hand raised to chest height, palm inward.

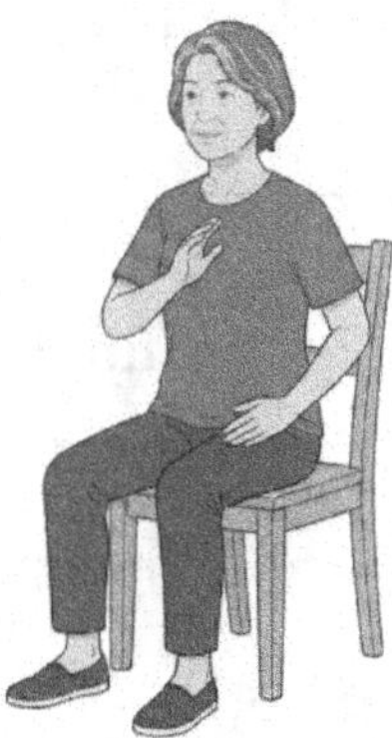

Steps:

1. Begin rotating the pelvis to the right in a gentle horizontal circle as the right hand sweeps forward and across to the left at chest height.

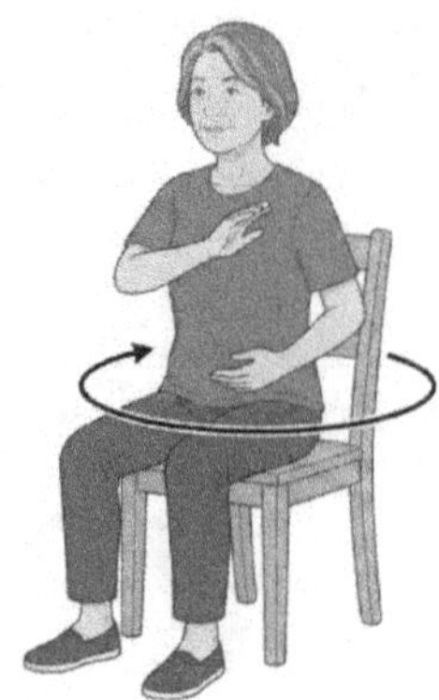

2. As the hip circle moves left, the left hand rises to chest height and sweeps across to the right, while the right hand descends to hip level.

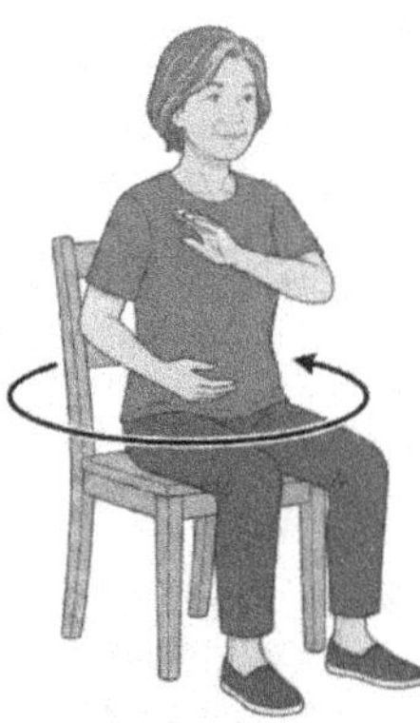

3. As the hip circle moves rearward, let the upper body follow the direction of the circle very slightly. The arms continue their alternating sweep.

4. Complete six full hip circles as the arms continue their continuous cloud-hands sweep.

5. Pause at center for one breath. Reverse the hip circle direction for six more repetitions.

BREATHING: Inhale as each hand rises. Exhale as it sweeps and descends. Let the hip circle follow the breath rather than being timed separately.

FEEL IT: A combined loosening through the hips and a continuous warmth in the arms. The coordination of hip circle and arm sweep becomes smoother over several sessions. In the first session, focus on one and let the other follow loosely.

IF NEEDED: Perform the hip circle and the arm sweep separately for the first few sessions if the coordination is difficult. When each is comfortable on its own, combine them.

Six circles each direction.

Form 7 – Waist Turn and Press

Trains the pushing strength of the arms and the rotational power of the waist together, building the core engagement that supports upright posture throughout the day.

Starting Position:

Sit in Tai Chi neutral. Right hand raised beside the right ear, palm facing forward. Left hand at hip level, palm facing downward.

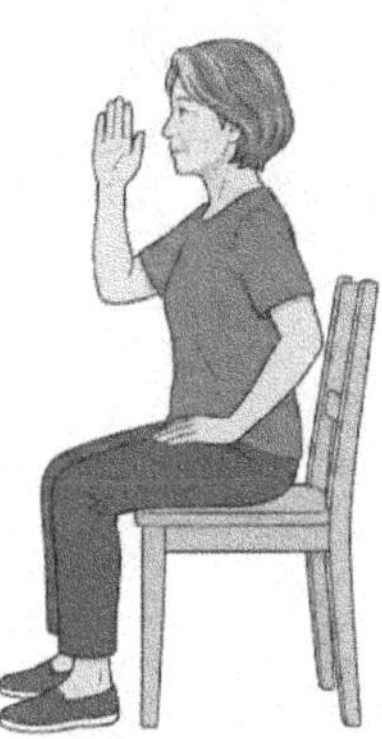

Steps:

1. Turn the upper body slightly to the right from the waist. Hips stay square to the front.
2. Begin pushing the right hand forward from beside the ear, palm leading, fingers pointing upward. Simultaneously sweep the left hand in a low arc across the front of the left hip from inside to outside.

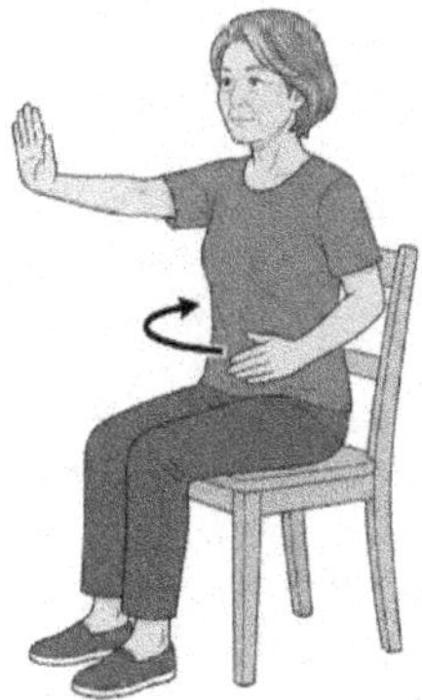

3. Hold the push position for one breath. Right arm extended forward, left hand at hip, upper body slightly turned right.

4. Return the upper body to center. Draw the right hand back beside the right ear. Reset the left hand at the right hip in preparation for the left-side repetition.

5. Turn left, push the left palm forward, sweep the right hand across the hip.

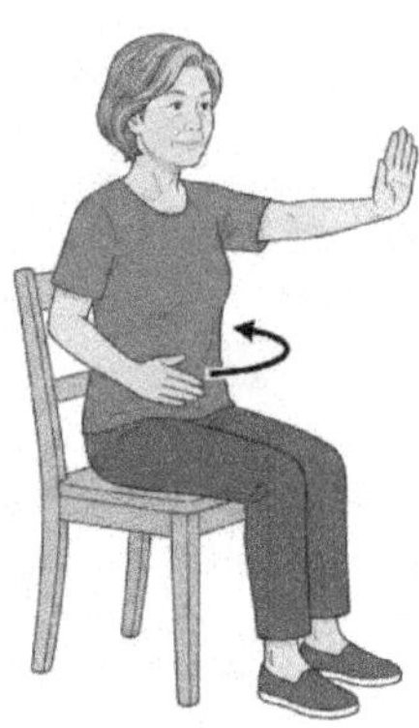

6. Complete four repetitions each side.

BREATHING: Inhale as you set up and turn. Exhale as the palm pushes forward.

FEEL IT: A clear engagement in the waist on the turning side and in the shoulder and upper arm on the pushing side. The push should feel as though it is powered by the waist turn, not by the arm alone.

IF NEEDED: Reduce the degree of waist turn if lower back discomfort is present. Even a small rotation produces the core engagement benefit.

Four repetitions each side.

Form 8 – Seated Closing Form

Completes every session. Signals to the nervous system and the practicing mind that the active portion is finished. Every session ends here, without exception.

Starting Position:

Sit in Tai Chi neutral after the final form of the session. Both hands resting in the lap.

Steps:

1. On a slow inhale, raise both arms forward to shoulder height, palms facing down, as though lifting something flat and light.

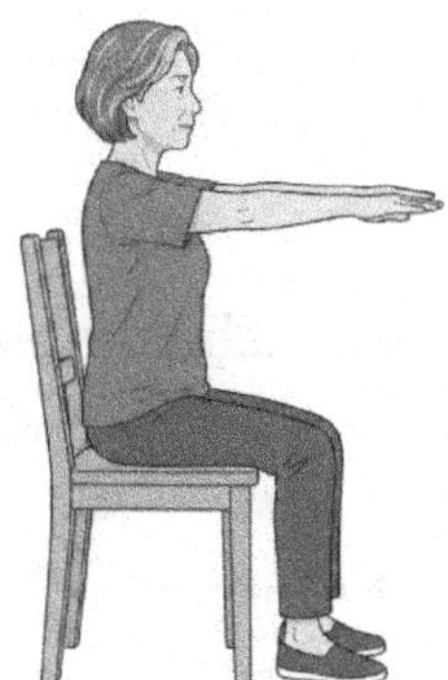

2. Pause at shoulder height for one full breath. Feel the chest wide and the spine long.

3. On the exhale, guide both arms back down slowly, palms angled toward the floor, letting them descend with weight and intention, not dropped, but lowered

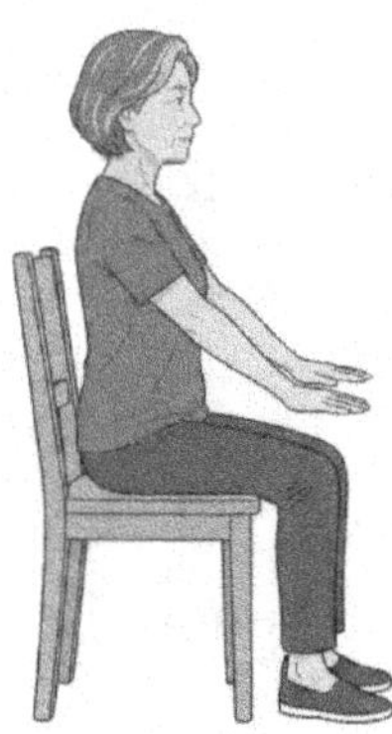

4. Bring both hands together in the lap, right hand over left, palms facing upward. Hold for three complete breaths.

5. On the third exhale, let everything settle. Notice the state of the body after practice.

BREATHING: Inhale as arms rise. Exhale as they lower. Three natural breaths for the final hold.

FEEL IT: A sense of completion. The breath returning to its resting rhythm. Some people notice a quieting of mental activity. Others notice warmth in the hands or a lightness in the shoulders. All are normal.

IF NEEDED: If raising the arms to full shoulder height is uncomfortable, raise to whatever height is manageable. The breath and the settling intention are the essential elements.

Every session ends with the Seated Closing Form.

Core and Posture Engagement

Every form in this chapter is built on a foundation of core engagement that the Sitting Tall exercise in Chapter Three began to establish. Understanding what the core is doing in the seated practice helps you do it better.

The core in seated Tai Chi is not the visible abdominal muscles. It is the deep stabilizers: the transversus abdominis, the multifidus along the spine, and the pelvic floor muscles. These muscles work continuously and quietly to maintain the Tai Chi neutral position throughout each session. They are muscles that most older adults have been activating deliberately, and their gradual strengthening through consistent practice produces changes that go beyond the practice itself.

A stronger deep core means a spine that requires less muscular effort to hold upright. Less effort means less fatigue. Less fatigue means more energy available for the forms themselves and for the rest of the day. Over several weeks, this effect compounds. People who have practiced consistently often report that sitting for extended periods becomes less uncomfortable, that lower back fatigue at the end of the day reduces, and that they find themselves sitting more upright in chairs generally, without thinking about it.

The deeper stabilizers also support the internal organs and contribute to the kind of intra-abdominal pressure management that protects the lower back during lifting, coughing, or any sudden movement. Strengthening them through seated Tai Chi practice therefore has benefits outside the session that many practitioners notice before they can name the cause.

The deliberate cue during any form where the core engagement slips is simply to return to the Sitting Tall position: press the feet into the floor, find the natural lumbar curve, lengthen the spine. These three actions re-engage the core automatically. They take less than two seconds and can be done at any point in any form without interrupting the movement.

Circulation Builders

These three movements are placed at the end of each session beginning in Week Three. They address circulation and lymphatic drainage specifically, targeting the structures most affected by prolonged sitting: the ankles, the knees, and the shoulder girdle. Done consistently after the main forms, they change how the body feels for the remainder of the day.

Circulation Builder 1 – Ankle Rolls

Activates the calf pump mechanism, improves venous return from the lower legs, and lubricates the ankle joints.

Starting Position:

Sit in Tai Chi neutral. Lift the right foot slightly off the floor, heel and toes both raised.

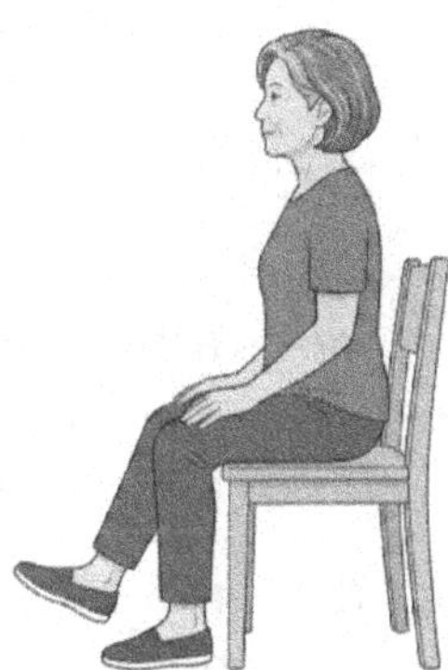

Steps:

1. Rotate the right ankle slowly in a full inward circle to the left side, five complete rotations. Keep the movement in the ankle, not the whole leg.

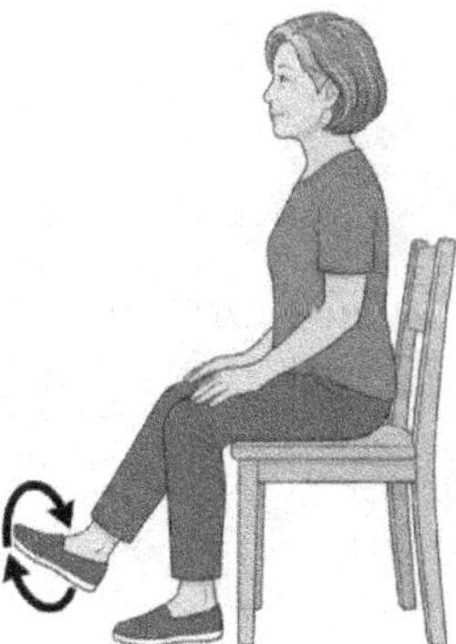

2. Reverse to five outward circles to the right side.
3. Lower the right foot. Lift the left foot and repeat: five inward, five outward.

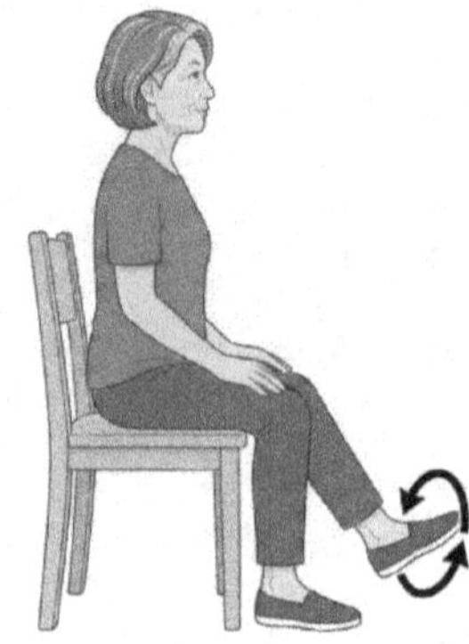

4. Lower the left foot. Press both feet flat into the floor and hold for one breath.

BREATHING: Breathe naturally throughout.

FEEL IT: A warmth and lightness in the ankles after the circles. If the feet have been cold or heavy, this usually resolves within two or three sets.

IF NEEDED: If lifting the foot causes hip discomfort, keep the heel on the floor and lift only the toes, rotating from there. Same ankle benefit, less hip load.

Circulation Builder 2 – Seated Knee Lifts

Activates the hip flexors and quadriceps, promotes lymphatic drainage from the thigh, and reinforces the seated postural stability that the forms require.

Starting Position:

Sit in Tai Chi neutral, both feet flat on the floor.

Steps:

1. Lift the right knee slowly upward, raising the right foot four to six inches off the floor. Keep the spine long and the pelvis level.

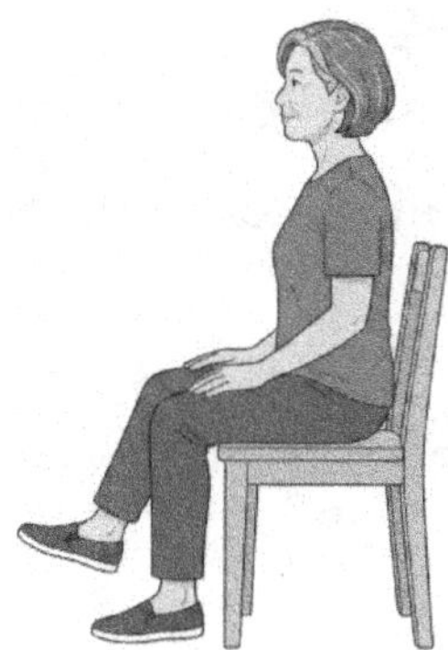

2. Hold for two counts at the top.

3. Lower the right foot slowly back to the floor.

4. Lift the left knee in the same way. Hold for two counts. Lower slowly.

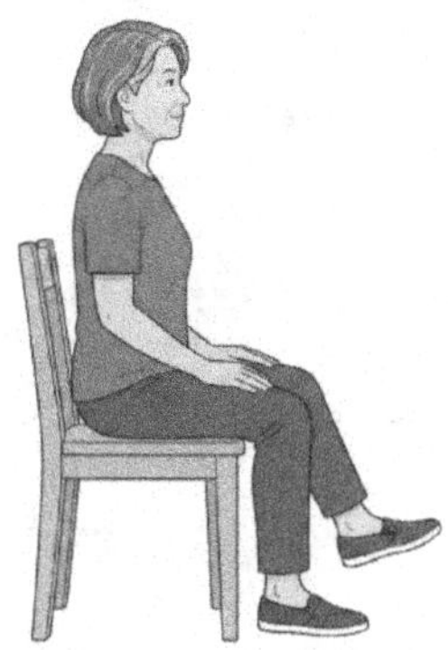

5. Alternate for 10 lifts each side. Complete and controlled pace.

BREATHING: Exhale as you lift. Inhale as you lower.

FEEL IT: A clear engagement in the front of the thigh on the lifting side. Some people also notice the deep abdominal muscles engaging to stabilize the pelvis during the lift.

IF NEEDED: Reduce the height of the lift if hip flexor tightness makes the full range uncomfortable. Even a small lift activates the target muscles.

10 lifts each side.

Circulation Builder 3 – Shoulder Rolls

Restores circulation to the upper back and shoulder girdle, releases the postural tension that accumulates during seated practice, and completes the session's work on the thoracic region.

Starting Position:

Sit in Tai Chi neutral, both hands resting on the thighs.

Steps:

1. Lift both shoulders upward toward the ears on a slow inhale.
2. Roll them backward and downward in a wide circle on the exhale. Five complete backward circles.

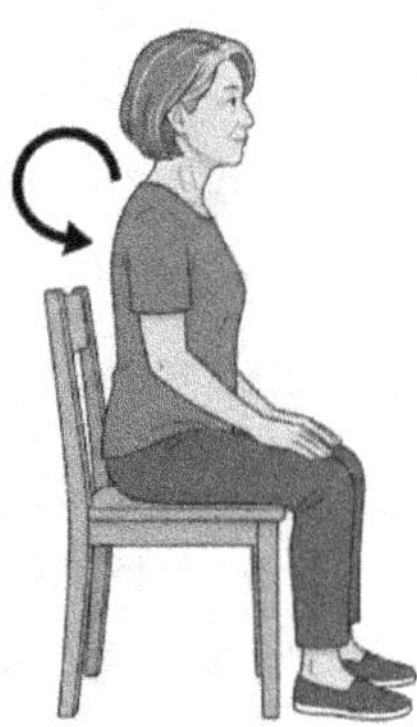

3. Reverse direction: roll the shoulders forward and upward, then downward. Five forward circles.
4. Let the shoulders settle in their lowest, most relaxed position. They should feel noticeably lower and softer than when you began.

BREATHING: Inhale as shoulders rise. Exhale as they roll down and back.

FEEL IT: A release of accumulated tension in the upper trapezius and across the top of the shoulders. Many people notice this is where they carry most of their held tension, and that five circles resolves most of it.

IF NEEDED: Reduce the size of the circle if shoulder clicking or pinching occurs. Even small rolls produce the circulation benefit.

Five circles each direction.

A Small Request

If working through this book has done something useful for you even one small thing that shifted, it would mean a great deal to hear about it. Would you be willing to leave a short, honest review on Amazon?

As an independent author, books like this one find their readers through honest reviews not advertising, not algorithms, just one person telling another that something helped them. If the past 4 chapters read so far produced any change you would want someone else to know about, a short review on Amazon is the most direct way to pass that along.

Two minutes. One or two sentences. That is genuinely all it takes, and it matters more than most people realize.

You can leave your review on Amazon by searching the title ***Chair Tai Chi for Weight Loss by Jing Weston*** on Amazon. It takes two minutes, and it matters more than you know.

Chapter 5

The 28-Day Program

Open this chapter each morning, find your day, and follow the session. Everything you need is on the page in front of you. The movement instructions are in Chapter Four.

Two things are worth holding before you begin. First: consistency matters more than quality of execution. A session done imperfectly is worth more than one skipped while waiting to feel ready. Second: the rest days are not empty. They are built into the program deliberately. The body adapts during recovery, not during effort. Honor them.

Week 1 – Settle In

This week is three forms, one breathing practice, and ten minutes a day. No more. The sessions are short because they are meant to be completed, not survived. Cloud Hands, Dragon Stirs the Waters, and Lotus Arms are the forms for the week. You will add nothing until Week Two.

The awkwardness of the first two sessions is normal and expected. The nervous system is registering new movement patterns. By Day 5 the forms will feel more like something the body already knows. That shift is the point of Week One.

The breathing practice that begins every session is not a warm-up. It is the practice itself, beginning. Six cycles of diaphragmatic breath before the first form lowers cortisol, activates the parasympathetic nervous system, and brings the practitioner into the quality of attention the forms require. Do not rush past it to get to the movements. The breath is the first movement.

What You Might Feel This Week
• Your hips and shoulder may feel stiff in the first session — especially if you have been sitting for long stretches. Give it two or three minutes of movement. It nearly always loosens

> • After you finish and sit quietly at the end of the Seated Closing Form, notice how your body
> feels. Most people describe something between calm and clear. It usually arrives by Day 2 or
> 3 if it is not felt on Day 1
> • Expect some fatigue in the muscles around your deep back and hips after Days 2 and 3. That
> is the seated posture waking up those muscles.

Your Win This Week: Your only target this week is the chair. Sit down, start the breathing practice, and do the forms. It does not matter whether you do them well. It matters that you do them. Seven days from now you will be glad you did not wait until you felt ready.

Day 1 – First Contact

SESSION AT A GLANCE
Duration: 10 minutes
Breathing Practice (Ch. 3): 6 cycles
Form 1: Seated Cloud Hands: 8 cycles
Form 2: Dragon Stirs the Waters: 5 circles each direction
Form 8: Seated Closing Form
Low energy: Breathing Practice + Closing Form only, 3 minutes

Jing's Note:
Day 1 asks only one thing of you: that you sit in the chair and begin. The forms do not need to be done well today. They do not need to look like the images. They need to be done.

NOTICE TODAY: After the Closing Form, sit still for one full breath. What does your body feel like compared to when you started?

Day 2 – Second Time

SESSION AT A GLANCE
Duration: 10 minutes
Breathing Practice: 6 cycles
Form 1: Seated Cloud Hands: 8 cycles
Form 2: Dragon Stirs the Waters: 5 circles each direction
Form 8: Seated Closing Form

Low energy: Breathing Practice + Closing Form only, 3 minutes

Jing's Note:
The second session is usually where people notice something they missed entirely on Day 1. Often it is in the breath. Notice whether the belly moves outward on the inhale today.

NOTICE TODAY: Does Cloud Hands feel different from yesterday? Even slightly?

Day 3 – Third Form

SESSION AT A GLANCE
Duration: 10 minutes

Breathing Practice: 6 cycles

Form 1: Seated Cloud Hands: 8 cycles

Form 2: Dragon Stirs the Waters: 5 circles each direction

Form 3: Lotus Arms: 6 repetitions

Form 8: Seated Closing Form

Low energy: Breathing Practice + Closing Form only, 3 minutes

Jing's Note:
Lotus Arms joins the sequence today. Three forms now. This is the full Week One practice. If the session runs a few minutes over while you find the pace, that is fine.

NOTICE TODAY: Which of the three forms feels least settled? That one deserves extra attention on Days 5 and 6.

Day 4 – Rest

REST DAY
No session today, that is intentional. Your body is still working, just differently. The muscles you have been engaging (deep back or lower spine, and hip muscles) are repairing and strengthening during this downtime. If anything feels a little stiff or heavy, that is a good sign. It means the practice is asking something real of you.

Day 5 – Return

SESSION AT A GLANCE

Duration: 10 minutes

Breathing Practice: 6 cycles

Form 1: Seated Cloud Hands: 8 cycles

Form 2: Dragon Stirs the Waters: 5 circles each direction

Form 3: Lotus Arms: 6 repetitions

Form 8: Seated Closing Form

Low energy: Breathing Practice + Closing Form only, 3 minutes

Jing's Note:

fIf this session feels slightly more settled than Day 3, that is not your imagination. Rest days are when the nervous system files what it has learned. The forms you practiced before the break are more organized now than they were when you stopped. Notice the difference

NOTICE TODAY: Does anything feel more natural today than it did on Day 3?

Day 6 – Longer Cloud Hands

SESSION AT A GLANCE

Duration: 10 minutes

Breathing Practice: 6 cycles

Form 1: Seated Cloud Hands: 10 cycles

Form 2: Dragon Stirs the Waters: 5 circles each direction

Form 3: Lotus Arms: 6 repetitions

Form 8: Seated Closing Form

Low energy: Breathing Practice + Closing Form only, 3 minutes

Jing's Note:

Cloud Hands increases to 10 cycles today. The additional time in the weight-shift deepens the hip engagement. Slow down slightly to stay within the session window.

NOTICE TODAY: Does the weight shift through the hips feel different at cycle 9 and 10 compared to cycle 1?

Day 7 – Rest

REST DAY

No practice today. Rest is not the opposite of progress — it is part of how progress happens. While you sit still today, your nervous system is organizing the movement patterns you have been building. Come back tomorrow. The forms will feel more like yours than they did before you stopped.

What to Expect This Week

The sessions in Week One are deliberately short, and this brevity is intentional rather than gradual. A ten-minute session completed every day produces more physiological benefit than a 30-minute session completed twice a week, for the reasons Chapter Two explains. The cortisol reduction from diaphragmatic breathing requires daily repetition to shift the baseline. The muscle activation patterns that the forms are establishing in the motor cortex need frequent reinforcement. Consistency of presence matters more than duration of effort.

Two things tend to surprise people in Week One. First: ten minutes is more than enough to feel a shift, not a dramatic one, but something real and quiet. Second: the Seated Closing Form, which looks like almost nothing on paper, is usually the part of the session that lands hardest. The few moments of stillness after deliberate movement turn out to be where the practice actually arrives.

What Week One does not produce is visible change on a scale or in the mirror. That is not what it is for. Week One is the nervous system learning the forms and the body learning the habit of showing up. The metabolic changes that follow later depend entirely on this foundation being laid first. Give this week its due and the weeks that follow will be built on solid ground.

Rest and Recovery

Rest days in this program are not wasted days. This program includes two rest days each week, which is especially important for seniors. The body adapts to new movement patterns primarily during sleep and rest, not during the sessions themselves. A session provides the stimulus. The rest day is where the nervous system consolidates the new motor patterns, where the postural muscles recover from sustained novel engagement, and where the hormonal changes produced by the breathing practice stabilize at a new baseline.

If you skipped a session during Week One and want to make it up, do not. Do not add an extra session on a rest day. Do not double up. The program is structured the way it is because the timing matters. What looks like a missed opportunity is simply the program running as designed.

Week 2 – Find Your Flow

Week Two adds Seated Single Whip and Gathering the Sky, bringing the total to five forms. Sessions increase to 12 minutes. Something that was not possible in Week One begins to happen: the forms start connecting. Instead of a list of separate exercises, a continuous thread begins to emerge.

Week Two is usually when the practice begins to make sense in a way Week One could not. With five forms now in the sequence, there is enough material to feel the thread running between them and that thread is what Tai Chi actually is.

> **What You Might Feel This Week**
> • The Week One forms will feel more settled, almost automatic by mid-week. This is exactly right. Let them run on their own rhythm.
> • Seated Single Whip requires a sustained arm extension. The shoulder girdle will notice this. That engagement is the point.
> • The 12-minute sessions will feel longer for the first two days. By Day 12 they will feel like the right length.

Your Win This Week: Link all five forms into one continuous sequence without

Day 8 – Fourth Form

> **SESSION AT A GLANCE**
> Duration: 12 minutes
> Breathing Practice: 6 cycles
> Forms 1-3 (Week One sequence)
> Form 4: Seated Single Whip: 3 reps each side
> Form 8: Seated Closing Form
> Low energy: Breathing Practice + Closing Form only, 3 minutes

> **Jing's Note:**

Seated Single Whip joins the sequence. The extended arm position asks more of the shoulder girdle than the Week One forms. Give it extra attention today. The transitions between forms are rough this week, and that is where they should be.

NOTICE TODAY: Which direction of Single Whip feels more stable: left arm extended or right arm extended?

Day 9 – Fifth Form

SESSION AT A GLANCE
Duration: 12 minutes

Breathing Practice: 6 cycles

Forms 1-4

Form 5: Gathering the Sky: 6 repetitions

Form 8: Seated Closing Form

Low energy: Breathing Practice + Closing Form only, 3 minutes

Jing's Note:
Gathering the Sky is the most vertical form in the practice. The overhead reach decompresses the spine in a way none of the other forms do. Notice what the lower back feels like at the top of the reach.

NOTICE TODAY: Does the overhead reach feel restricted at the shoulders, comfortable, or somewhere between?

Day 10 – Settling

SESSION AT A GLANCE
Duration: 12 minutes

Breathing Practice: 6 cycles

Forms 1-5 in sequence

Form 8: Seated Closing Form

Low energy: Breathing Practice + Closing Form only, 3 minutes

Jing's Note:

Five forms today as a full sequence. The pace determines whether you finish in 12 minutes. Slower forms are better forms. If time runs over slightly, reduce repetition counts rather than rushing.

NOTICE TODAY: Where does the flow break between forms? That transition is worth practicing separately before tomorrow.

Day 11 – Rest

REST DAY
No session today, that is intentional. Your body is still working, just differently. The muscles you have been engaging (deep back or lower spine, and hip muscles) are repairing and strengthening during this downtime. If anything feels a little stiff or heavy, that is a good sign. It means the practice is asking something real of you.

Day 12 – Extended Hip Work

SESSION AT A GLANCE
Duration: 12 minutes

Breathing Practice: 6 cycles

Form 1: Cloud Hands: 10 cycles

Form 2: Dragon Stirs the Waters: 7 circles each direction

Forms 3-5

Form 8: Seated Closing Form

Low energy: Breathing Practice + Closing Form only, 3 minutes

Jing's Note:
Dragon Stirs the Waters increases to seven circles each direction today. The additional time in the hip circle produces a deeper lubrication effect in the hip joints. You may feel the difference most clearly when standing up from the chair after the session.

NOTICE TODAY: Does the hip circle feel different in the seventh cycle compared to the first?

Day 13 – Consolidate

SESSION AT A GLANCE
Duration: 12 minutes

Breathing Practice: 6 cycles

Forms 1-5 with increased reps: Cloud Hands 10 cycles, Lotus Arms 8 reps, Gathering the Sky 8 reps

Form 8: Seated Closing Form

Low energy: Breathing Practice + Closing Form only, 3 minutes

Jing's Note:
Two weeks in. The check below is an observation, not a grade. Answer it honestly and carry what you learn into Week Three.

NOTICE TODAY: Return to the four baseline measures from Chapter Three. Compare where you are today.

PROGRESS CHECK

Take two minutes with these questions. Write the answers if you can.

Seated Reach: Does your forward reach extend further than on assessment day? ☐ Further ☐ Same ☐ Not sure

Hip Rotation: Does either direction of upper-body rotation feel more open? ☐ Yes ☐ About the same ☐ Not sure

Morning stiffness: Is it resolving more quickly than at the start? ☐ Yes ☐ About the same ☐ Variable

Energy rating: Rate your typical morning energy this past week on the same 1-5 scale. Write the number.

Sessions completed: How many of the 12 practice days did you complete? Write the number.

Week Three introduces all eight forms and the first Circulation Builder. Sessions increase to 15 minutes. If the five-form sequence still feels unsteady, continue practicing it at the start of each Week Three session before adding the new material.

Day 14 – Rest

REST DAY
No practice today. Rest is not the opposite of progress — it is part of how progress happens. While you sit still today, your nervous system is organizing the movement patterns you have been building. Come back tomorrow. The forms will feel more like yours than they did before you stopped.

Increasing Smoothness, Not Speed

Week Two is where things start to click. In Week One, just keeping up with the steps and getting the movements done takes everything you have got. By Week Two, your body has started to remember and because it is doing more of the work on its own, your mind gets to do something more useful: by actually feeling what is happening. If the weight is sitting evenly in the pelvis when you move through "Cloud Hands," or if it is sneaking to one side. If the hip circle in "Dragon Stirs the Waters" is staying flat and level the way it should, or if it is tilting. If the spine is genuinely lengthening, or the arms are just going up while everything below stays compressed when you reach up in "Gathering the Sky"

These are not complicated things to notice. But noticing them is exactly what moves the practice forward. Seated Tai Chi does not get better by speeding up. It gets better by paying closer attention. Week Two is the first week where that distinction becomes practically available.

The temptation in Week Two is to pick up the pace. Resist it. Speed does not make this practice more effective, it makes it a different practice, and not a better one. Everything that gives seated Tai Chi its physiological value, the breath coordination, the joint lubrication, the sustained muscle engagement, depends on the pace staying slow enough for the breath to lead. If you are moving faster than your exhale, pull back. That is always the right adjustment.

Week 3 – Turn Up the Work

Week Three completes the form set. Hip Circle Flow, Waist Turn and Press, and the Seated Closing Form as a formal closing ritual all join the sequence. The first Circulation Builder appears at the end of sessions. Sessions increase to 15 minutes.

Week Three is where the groundwork laid in the first two weeks starts to pay off in a way you can actually feel. The breathing practice has been quietly lowering your baseline cortisol since Day One. The eight forms have been reactivating muscles that sedentary sitting had switched off. By this week, both of those processes are running together and most people notice the difference in their energy somewhere around Day 17 or 18.

> **What You Might Feel This Week**

- Hip Circle Flow and Waist Turn and Press require simultaneous hip and arm coordination. In the first two sessions they will feel uncoordinated. That is normal and resolves by Day 18.
- Ankle Rolls, the first Circulation Builder, produce a warmth and lightness in the lower legs that many people have not felt in years.
- Some people notice clearer sleep around Day 16 to 18. This is the cortisol regulation effect accumulating.

Your Win This Week: Complete the full eight-form sequence, including all three new forms, at least twice.

Day 15 – Sixth Form

SESSION AT A GLANCE
Duration: 15 minutes
Breathing Practice: 6 cycles
Forms 1-5
Form 6: Hip Circle Flow: 6 circles each direction
Form 8: Seated Closing Form
Low energy: Breathing Practice + Closing Form only, 3 minutes

Jing's Note:
Hip Circle Flow combines the hip rotation from Dragon Stirs the Waters with the arm sweep from Cloud Hands. In the first session, focus on the hip circle and let the arms follow loosely. The coordination comes with repetition.

NOTICE TODAY: Does the hip circle feel different when the arms are moving simultaneously versus in isolation?

Day 16 – Seventh Form

SESSION AT A GLANCE
Duration: 15 minutes
Breathing Practice: 6 cycles
Forms 1-6
Form 7: Waist Turn and Press: 4 reps each side
Form 8: Seated Closing Form
Low energy: Breathing Practice + Closing Form only, 3 minutes

Jing's Note:
Waist Turn and Press asks the waist to power the arm push, not the shoulder. In the first session, most people use the shoulder. By Day 20 most people have found the waist.

NOTICE TODAY: Can you feel the waist engaging on the push, or does it feel like a shoulder movement?

Day 17 – Circulation Builder

SESSION AT A GLANCE
Duration: 15 minutes
Breathing Practice: 6 cycles
Full eight-form sequence
Circulation Builder 1: Ankle Rolls (Ch. 4): 5 circles each ankle each direction
Form 8: Seated Closing Form
Low energy: Breathing Practice + Closing Form only, 3 minutes

Jing's Note:
The first Circulation Builder joins the session today. Ankle Rolls after the main forms. Five circles each direction on each ankle. The legs may feel noticeably lighter afterward.

NOTICE TODAY: What does the lower leg feel like after the ankle rolls compared to before them?

Day 18 – Rest

REST DAY
No practice today. Rest is not the opposite of progress — it is part of how progress happens. While you sit still today, your nervous system is organizing the movement patterns you have been building. Come back tomorrow. The forms will feel more like yours than they did before you stopped.

Day 19 – Waist Focus

SESSION AT A GLANCE
Duration: 15 minutes
Breathing Practice: 6 cycles

Full eight-form sequence with focus on Forms 6 and 7

Circulation Builder 1: Ankle Rolls

Form 8: Seated Closing Form

Low energy: Breathing Practice + Closing Form only, 3 minutes

Jing's Note:
Give Forms 6 and 7 particular attention today. After four sessions, the coordination of hip and arm in Hip Circle Flow should be starting to settle. Check whether the waist is driving Waist Turn and Press.

NOTICE TODAY: In Waist Turn and Press: does the push feel stronger when the waist turns first?

Day 20 – Continuous Eight

SESSION AT A GLANCE
Duration: 15 minutes

Breathing Practice: 6 cycles

Full eight-form sequence, continuous if possible

Circulation Builder 1: Ankle Rolls

Form 8: Seated Closing Form

Low energy: Breathing Practice + Closing Form only, 3 minutes

Jing's Note:
No form-by-form breakdown today. Run all eight forms in one unbroken sequence. When you need to find your next movement, use the breath as the bridge. One complete breath between forms gives you just enough time to locate where you are without breaking the flow. If something goes wrong, come back to Cloud Hands and pick up from there.

NOTICE TODAY: How far through the continuous sequence did you get before needing to redirect?

PROGRESS CHECK
Three weeks of practice. Answer honestly.

Seated Reach: Compare to Day 13 check and to original baseline. □ Further than Day 13 □ Same □ Variable

Hip Rotation: Is either direction more open than at Day 13? □ More open □ Same □ Not sure

Breath hold comfortable pause: Count again. Compare to baseline. ☐ Longer ☐ Same ☐ Shorter on tired days

Energy rating: Rate your typical morning energy this week on the same 1-5 scale. Write the number.

Can you complete the full eight-form sequence without stopping? ☐ Yes ☐ With one or two pauses ☐ Still building

Week Four brings the complete practice together: all eight forms and two Circulation Builders. Sessions increase to 15 to 20 minutes. This is the week where the practice begins to feel like it belongs to you.

Day 21 – Rest

REST DAY

No session today, that is intentional. Your body is still working, just differently. The muscles you have been engaging (deep back or lower spine, and hip muscles) are repairing and strengthening during this downtime. If anything feels a little stiff or heavy, that is a good sign. It means the practice is asking something real of you.

Building Real Strength Without Strain

The eight-form sequence, practiced daily, produces a specific pattern of muscular adaptation. The deep stabilizers of the spine and hips strengthen through the sustained postural demand of every session. The shoulder girdle builds endurance through the repeated arm movements of Cloud Hands, Lotus Arms, Seated Single Whip, and Gathering the Sky. The hip rotators develop both flexibility and strength through Dragon Stirs the Waters and Hip Circle Flow. The core builds through every moment the spine is held long.

This is not dramatic strength development. It is the gradual rebuilding of functional capacity that sedentary living erodes: the ability to hold the body upright without fatigue, to rotate the hips through their full range, to carry the arms through sustained movement without the shoulders tiring. These are the capacities that make daily life easier and fall risk lower. They are built by exactly the kind of slow, deliberate, sustained movement this practice provides.

Where Fat Burn Shifts Up a Gear

Three weeks of consistent diaphragmatic breathing practice produces measurable cortisol reduction that is now persistent rather than session-specific. In the first week, cortisol drops during and for several hours after each session. By Week Three, the resting baseline itself has begun to shift. The hormonal environment that drives abdominal fat storage is less consistently present. This is the turning point that the first two weeks were building toward.

By the time you reach Week Three, something has already shifted — you just may not have noticed it yet. The cortisol reduction from your daily breathing practice has been building since Day One. The muscle activation patterns the forms are establishing have been telling the nervous system to keep those pathways alive. Now, in Week Three, these two threads begin working in the same direction at the same time. What that means in practice: the hormonal environment that drives abdominal fat storage is less consistently active. The muscles that support your resting metabolic rate are being asked to stay switched on rather than going dormant. None of this shows up on a scale in Week Three. It shows up later. But the work is happening now, underneath whatever you can see

Week 4 – Own the Practice

The final week adds a second Circulation Builder: Seated Knee Lifts. Sessions increase to 15 to 20 minutes. Everything else holds: the same eight forms, the same breathing practice, the Seated Closing Form at the end.

Week Four is when the practice becomes self-sustaining for most people. The forms are familiar enough that the mental effort of following instructions drops away. What remains is the practice itself.

Two Circulation Builders in Week Four add approximately four minutes to each session. This brings the full practice to 15 to 20 minutes. For people who found 10 minutes easy, 20 minutes is an appropriate challenge. For people who found 10 minutes sufficient, 15 minutes is a reasonable target. The session length is a guide, not a requirement. Complete the forms and both Circulation Builders at whatever pace allows full attention and correct posture throughout.

What You Might Feel This Week

• Running through all eight forms should start to feel like one thing rather than eight separate things. The mental effort of organizing the sequence has dropped. What is left is the practice itself and that is a different experience than what Week One felt like

• Seated Knee Lifts will produce a clear engagement in the front of the thighs and deep core. That engagement is the point.

> • Some people feel, around Day 25 or 26, a specific quality of quiet after the Seated Closing Form that is different from any earlier point in the program.

Your Win This Week: Complete the full practice, all eight forms and both Circulation Builders, on every practice day.

Day 22 – Two Builders

SESSION AT A GLANCE
Duration: 15-20 minutes
Breathing Practice: 6 cycles
Full eight-form sequence
Circulation Builder 1: Ankle Rolls
Circulation Builder 2: Seated Knee Lifts (Ch. 4): 10 lifts each side
Form 8: Seated Closing Form
Low energy: Breathing Practice + Closing Form only, 3 minutes

Jing's Note:
Seated Knee Lifts join the sequence. Ten lifts each side after Ankle Rolls. Both Circulation Builders together take about four minutes. The legs will notice them.

NOTICE TODAY: What do the thighs feel like during the knee lifts? A clear engagement or something more diffuse?

Day 23 – Full Practice

SESSION AT A GLANCE
Duration: 15-20 minutes
Breathing Practice: 6 cycles
Full eight-form sequence
Circulation Builders 1 and 2
Form 8: Seated Closing Form
Low energy: Breathing Practice + Closing Form only, 3 minutes

Jing's Note:

This is the complete Week Four practice. The full session, all elements in sequence. Twenty minutes when done at full pace. Note how different 20 minutes feels from the 10 minutes of Day 1.

NOTICE TODAY: How does the body feel at the end of 20 minutes compared to how it felt at the end of 10 minutes in Week One?

Day 24 – Rest

REST DAY
No practice today. Rest is not the opposite of progress — it is part of how progress happens. While you sit still today, your nervous system is organizing the movement patterns you have been building. Come back tomorrow. The forms will feel more like yours than they did before you stopped.

Day 25 – Extended Knee Lifts

SESSION AT A GLANCE
Duration: 15-20 minutes
Breathing Practice: 6 cycles
Full eight-form sequence
Circulation Builder 1: Ankle Rolls
Circulation Builder 2: Seated Knee Lifts: 12 lifts each side
Form 8: Seated Closing Form
Low energy: Breathing Practice + Closing Form only, 3 minutes

Jing's Note:
Knee lifts increase to 12 each side today. The additional reps extend the time the hip flexors and quadriceps are working. The carryover into standing and walking is usually noticeable.

NOTICE TODAY: What feels different in the legs at the end of 12 lifts compared to the end of 10?

Day 26 – Last Full Session

SESSION AT A GLANCE
Duration: 15-20 minutes

Breathing Practice: 6 cycles

Full eight-form sequence

Circulation Builders 1 and 2 at full reps

Form 8: Seated Closing Form

Low energy: Breathing Practice + Closing Form only, 3 minutes

Jing's Note:
The last full practice day before the final check. Do the session as you have been doing it. The ceremony is in having shown up consistently.

NOTICE TODAY: What part of the practice do you find yourself looking forward to? The answer is usually interesting.

Day 27 – Rest

REST DAY
No practice today. Rest is not the opposite of progress — it is part of how progress happens. While you sit still today, your nervous system is organizing the movement patterns you have been building. Come back tomorrow. The forms will feel more like yours than they did before you stopped.

Day 28 – Final Day

SESSION AT A GLANCE
Duration: 15-20 minutes

Breathing Practice: 6 cycles

Full eight-form sequence, continuous

Circulation Builders 1 and 2

Form 8: Seated Closing Form. Hold the final stillness for five full breaths.

Jing's Note:
Twenty-eight days. Hold the Seated Closing Form longer today. Five full breaths in the final position. Let the practice land before you do the check below.

NOTICE TODAY: Return to every measure from Chapter Three and from both progress checks. Read your earlier answers. Then answer them now.

PROGRESS CHECK

Putting the Full Flow Together

The final week is where the practice first feels like a single coherent thing rather than a sequence of separate exercises. The breath has been coordinating with the movement long enough that it happens without deliberate direction. The transitions between forms have been practiced enough that the brain no longer has to hunt for the next movement. What is left, in the space that careful instruction previously occupied, is actual practice.

This is what Tai Chi practitioners describe when they talk about the practice becoming their own. Not mastery. Not the absence of imperfection. The presence of the practitioner in the movement rather than the movement as a task being performed. Twenty-eight days is enough to arrive at the edge of that quality. A few more weeks of consistent practice moves the practitioner clearly inside it.

Feeling Better in the Chair and Beyond

The phrase 'No Standing Required' in this book's title is not a consolation. It is a description of a complete practice. Every mechanism by which seated Tai Chi produces its results, cortisol reduction through diaphragmatic breath, muscle activation through sustained controlled movement, improved circulation through deliberate full-body engagement, operates fully from the chair. The outcomes described in the research on seated Tai Chi for older adults are not qualified by posture. They are produced by the practice, and the practice is performed seated.

What standing Tai Chi has over seated practice is the additional challenge of managing dynamic balance. What seated Tai Chi has over standing practice is accessibility to people for whom that challenge is not yet safe or appropriate. These are different practices with different applications. This book is the seated version, and it is complete in itself.

By the end of Day 28, most people have a version of the complete practice that is genuinely their own. Not perfect. But functional, consistent, and no longer a program being followed. The forms have become a sequence the body knows.

The scale may not have moved dramatically. For many people it moves modestly. For some it has not moved at all, while body composition has shifted in ways that the scale does not capture. Muscle gained during the program displaces fat lost on the scale measurement, producing the frustrating result of identical numbers describing a genuinely different body. The instruction at this point is always the same: set the scale aside for six weeks and continue practicing. The changes that 28 days began take several more weeks to register on a measure as blunt as total body mass.

The changes that 28 days of consistent seated practice produces are specific. Cortisol is lower as a baseline. The hip joints move more freely. The deep core stabilizers are stronger and more reliably engaged. Sleep is, for most practitioners, measurably better. Circulation in the lower legs has improved. The seated posture is more upright and less effortful. These are real changes. They compound with continued practice. The 28-day program did not produce them in full. It started them.

Chapter 6

Fueling the Work

No calorie counting. No food rules. No weekly meal plan. This chapter is not that kind of nutrition guidance. What it offers instead is a small set of eating principles that directly support what the seated practice is building in your body. Simple, practical, and grounded in how the physiology of this particular program actually works.

Movement Without Punishment

The conventional weight loss model pairs exercise with restriction. Move more, eat less. For many older adults, this pairing has been tried before and has produced a familiar cycle: initial progress, diminishing returns, fatigue, and eventual abandonment of both the exercise and the dietary change.

This approach takes a different position. The practice you have built over 28 days is itself a physiological intervention. It is lowering cortisol, improving insulin sensitivity, activating muscle tissue, and improving sleep quality. Each of these changes shifts the body toward a state where fat loss becomes progressively more possible. Adding aggressive caloric restriction on top of this process undermines it. The body reads a significant combined calorie and energy deficit as a threat and responds by protecting its fat stores more conservatively, reducing resting metabolic rate, and increasing cravings for high-calorie foods. The net result is often less progress than the practice alone would produce.

The instruction, then, is this: do not diet while you practice. Make the two or three specific adjustments described in this chapter, which support the practice directly without adding significant restriction, and leave everything else roughly as it has been. Once the movement habit is established and the body has adapted, the nutritional refinements can happen incrementally, one at a time, with the bandwidth to give them proper attention.

Food is not a punishment for having a body. It is fuel for the work. This chapter is about matching the fuel to what the work actually needs.

One practical note: people who have tried restrictive eating approaches in the past sometimes find that even thinking about food in terms of what to eat produces a stress response. If that is the case, read this chapter as permission rather than instruction. The suggestions here are not requirements. They are options that tend to work well for people doing this practice. Take the ones that feel accessible. Leave the ones that do not. Come back to the others when the practice is more established and the bandwidth exists.

What to Eat More Of

Rather than a list of restrictions, this chapter offers additions. These are the foods and eating patterns that directly support the physiological changes the practice is producing.

Protein at every meal.

Muscle tissue is built and maintained from dietary protein. As the seated forms rebuild the deep stabilizers and the postural muscles, the body needs available amino acids to do that rebuilding. Most older adults consume less protein than their bodies require to maintain muscle mass, and a deficit slows the muscle preservation that keeps resting metabolic rate elevated.

The practical target is roughly half a gram of protein per pound of body weight per day. For a 150-pound person, that is about 75 grams. Spread across three meals, that is 25 grams per meal, which is two eggs plus Greek yogurt at breakfast, a palm-sized serving of fish or chicken at lunch, and a similar serving at dinner. No protein powder required. No dramatic change to eating patterns. Just consistent attention to including a protein source at each meal.

Anti-inflammatory foods.

The practice lowers systemic inflammation through cortisol reduction and improved circulation. Certain foods amplify this effect. Fatty fish such as salmon, mackerel, and sardines eaten two or three times per week provide omega-3 fatty acids that directly reduce inflammatory markers. Berries, leafy greens, walnuts, olive oil, and turmeric all support the anti-inflammatory direction the practice is establishing. These are not medicine. They are food that works with what the practice is already doing.

Foods that work against the anti-inflammatory direction are the familiar ones: high-sugar processed foods, refined carbohydrates in large quantities, excessive alcohol. None of these needs to be permanently removed. Volume and frequency are what matter. A general trend in the useful direction, maintained consistently, produces the same cumulative benefit as a strict exclusion list maintained erratically.

Sufficient overall calories.

Undereating is as significant a problem as overeating for older adults doing a new movement practice. The body needs energy to support the metabolic activity the practice is producing. People who restrict calories significantly while beginning a movement program often feel fatigued, find the forms harder to concentrate on, and experience the frustrating outcome of burning muscle for fuel rather than fat. Eat enough to feel energized for the session. Hunger during practice is a signal that food was insufficient beforehand.

Adequate carbohydrate around sessions.

Seated Tai Chi is a sustained low-intensity activity that relies on fat oxidation as its primary fuel. However, the muscles also use glycogen, and sessions that follow periods of very low carbohydrate intake sometimes feel heavy and uncoordinated. A small carbohydrate-containing snack before the session, a piece of fruit, a few whole grain crackers, a small bowl of oatmeal, ensures the muscles have what they need to perform the forms with the control and coordination the practice depends on.

Timing Meals Around Sessions

When you practice relative to when you eat affects how the session feels and how effectively the body uses the practice's metabolic window.

Before practice.

Practicing on a completely empty stomach is manageable for some people and uncomfortable for others. A light snack 30 to 45 minutes before the session, small enough not to compete with the breathing practice but large enough to prevent the energy dip that some older adults experience during sustained seated concentration, serves most people well. A piece of fruit, a small handful of nuts, a single hard-boiled egg, or half a banana with a spoonful of nut butter. Nothing heavy. Nothing that produces digestive discomfort during the hip circles or waist turns.

After practice.

The increased insulin sensitivity that follows each session is real and time-limited. A protein-containing meal or snack within 30 to 60 minutes of the session's end routes glucose into muscle cells rather than into fat storage. This is the post-practice nutritional window that the physiology chapter described. A properly timed meal after the session converts the practice's metabolic benefit into muscle preservation rather than letting the window close unused.

The timing principle extends to the rest of the day as well. People who skip meals entirely, eating only once or twice daily, often find their sessions feel harder and their energy less stable. The body regulates appetite signals through insulin, cortisol, and leptin, all of which are affected by meal frequency. Three moderate meals each with protein, distributed through the day, keeps these signals more stable than two large meals with long gaps. This is an observation that tends to be useful for older adults doing a daily movement practice.

Practical after-practice meals: two eggs any style with vegetables. A bowl of Greek yogurt with fruit and a handful of walnuts. Canned salmon or tuna with whole grain crackers and cucumber. A serving of legume soup with whole grain bread. Cottage cheese with sliced fruit. Each takes under ten minutes to prepare and delivers the protein the muscles need within the window that matters.

Water, Rest, and the Quiet Drivers of Change

These three factors, hydration, sleep, and the accumulated rest the body needs to adapt to new movement patterns, drive more of the body's fat loss and body composition change than most people recognize. They work quietly and their effects are easy to attribute to other causes. But when they are missing, the practice underperforms.

Water.

Hydration is one of those things that does its work quietly in the background. You will not always feel the difference day to day but your joints will, your energy will, and the cortisol clearance that this practice depends on will. The kidneys need water to carry metabolic byproducts out of the body after each session. The synovial fluid that keeps your hip and spinal joints moving freely needs water to maintain its viscosity. A straightforward habit that helps: one glass before you sit down to practice, one glass after you finish. No tracking required. Just two glasses tied to something you are already doing. That small habit alone makes a real difference in how your legs feel and how fast that morning stiffness clears up.

Many older adults are chronically mildly dehydrated without knowing it. The thirst mechanism becomes less reliable with age. By the time thirst registers, mild dehydration has already affected energy, cognitive clarity, and joint comfort. Proactive hydration, drinking before the sensation of thirst, is particularly important for this population.

Sleep.

Every session you do is a signal to the body. Sleep is where the body answers it. During deep sleep, your muscles complete the repair that the forms began, cortisol clears from the system, and the hormones that regulate hunger and fat metabolism reset for the next day. Practicing daily while consistently short-sleeping is a bit like trying to fill a glass with a hole in it — the practice is working, but the overnight reset is not completing, so the gains accumulate more slowly than they should. Most adults need seven to eight hours for these processes to complete properly. If your typical night is consistently under six, that one variable may be doing more to slow your results than anything about the practice itself. And if it does not get finished, the progress the practice is building simply does not show up the way it should.

For most adults, anything less than seven hours starts to compromise the body's overnight recovery. Drop below six consistently and the consequences are measurable: the stress hormone does not fully clear, the hormone responsible for muscle repair is released in smaller amounts, and the signals that govern appetite shift toward craving rather than satisfaction. These are not background inconveniences. They are large enough to blunt the gains the practice is building during the day. Sleep is not a bonus on top of this program. It is part of the program.

The practice itself supports better sleep through its cortisol-lowering effect. This creates a positive cycle: better practice produces lower cortisol, lower cortisol produces better sleep, better sleep allows fuller recovery, fuller recovery produces better practice. Establishing this cycle is one of the most valuable things the 28-day program does. Protect it by keeping a consistent sleep and wake time, avoiding screens in the hour before bed, and treating adequate sleep as a component of the practice rather than a separate concern.

Coffee and tea are fine, both contribute to your daily fluid intake and do not need to be cut unless they are keeping you awake. Alcohol is a different matter. It dehydrates the body and interferes with the overnight cortisol clearance that this practice depends on. Cutting back in the evenings, even modestly, tends to produce a noticeable improvement in sleep quality and that improvement carries more weight here than any other single dietary adjustment.

Rest between sessions.

The rest days built into the program are not empty time. They are the days when the neural adaptations to new movement patterns consolidate, when the postural muscles recover from the sustained engagement of the forms, and when the hormonal shifts produced by each session stabilize into the new baseline. People who skip rest days in the first weeks of a new practice often feel better in the short term and worse in the third and fourth weeks, because the accumulated physical debt eventually demands payment.

Honor the rest days. Use them for gentle activity if desired, walking, stretching, the breathing practice alone. But honor them as recovery rather than opportunity for additional effort. The practice is built in the active sessions. The gains are made in the rest.

A body that moves daily, eats enough protein, drinks adequate water, and sleeps seven to eight hours has addressed every major lever available for healthy weight management at this stage of life. Not one of those levers requires a special product, a gym, or a standing exercise format. They require consistency and attention. The chair practice provides the movement. This chapter provides the nutritional context. The rest is yours to build.

Food is part of the practice, even when the practice is happening in a chair. The body that shows up to the session each morning is built from everything eaten in the days before.

The complete and practical summary: eat protein at every meal, include some anti-inflammatory foods most days, have a light snack before the session if the body needs it, eat a proper meal within an hour after, drink two glasses of water deliberately rather than waiting for thirst, protect sleep as though it is part of the practice, and honor the rest days. That is the complete nutritional support system for this program. None of it requires counting, tracking, or eliminating anything permanently.

Chapter 7

Strength and Mobility Beyond the Chair

The forms in Chapter Four are not contained to the chair. The strength, the postural habits, the hip mobility, the shoulder range, and the breath coordination they develop transfer directly into daily life. This chapter names where that transfer happens and offers four micro-movements that extend the practice into the hours between sessions.

What Seated Practice Builds That You Feel Everywhere

People who practice seated Tai Chi consistently for several weeks often describe changes in their daily life that they do not immediately attribute to the practice. They sit through a long meal without the lower back beginning to ache. They turn to look over their shoulder while driving and notice the rotation is easier. They stand up from a low sofa with less effort than before. These are not separate improvements. They are the direct transfer of what the practice has been building.

Core stability.

The deep stabilizers of the spine that the Tai Chi neutral seated position demands gradually become stronger and more reliably engaged. Over several weeks of daily practice, this engagement becomes the default rather than the deliberate choice. The body begins holding itself more upright automatically, in chairs outside the practice, in cars, at tables, anywhere it is seated. The lower back fatigue that many older adults experience after extended sitting reduces as the muscles that were previously uninvolved begin taking their share of the postural load.

This carries further than seated posture. The deep core stabilizers that support the spine while seated are the same muscles that control the trunk during walking, reaching, and bending. Stronger stabilizers mean more controlled movement across all of these activities. Falls often result from a trunk that cannot recover quickly from unexpected perturbation. The stabilizer strength built in ten minutes of daily seated practice directly addresses this vulnerability.

Hip mobility.

Dragon Stirs the Waters and Hip Circle Flow move the hip joints through rotational ranges that most older adults' daily activity never includes. The hip rotators are among the first to weaken with inactivity, and their loss contributes to the shortened gait and forward lean that many older adults develop over time. Regular hip rotation through the forms restores both muscle function and joint range.

This hip mobility transfers directly to walking, stair climbing, and turning. People whose gait becomes more fluid after several weeks of practice are not imagining the connection.

Shoulder and upper back mobility.

Lotus Arms, Gathering the Sky, and Seated Single Whip move the shoulder joint through extension, elevation, and external rotation that seated daily life virtually never requires. The thoracic spine, which becomes progressively stiffer in people who sit in forward-flexed positions for extended periods, is mobilized through the rotation and extension demands of Waist Turn and Press and Hip Circle Flow. The combined effect is a shoulder girdle and upper back that can turn, reach overhead, and carry loads with less effort and less pain.

Four Daily Micro-Movements

These four movements take two minutes each and are designed for ordinary moments in the day: waiting for something to heat, sitting at a desk between tasks, pausing between activities. Done consistently outside the formal sessions, they maintain the mobility gains of the practice in the hours between sessions.

Micro-Movement 1 – Seated Spinal Rotation

Maintains thoracic mobility and waist rotation between sessions.

Starting Position:

Sit in Tai Chi neutral, feet flat on the floor, both hands resting on the thighs.

Steps:

1. Place both hands on the opposite thigh, left hand on right thigh, right hand on top of left.

2. On a slow exhale, rotate the upper body to the right, leading with the right shoulder. Keep the hips square to the front.

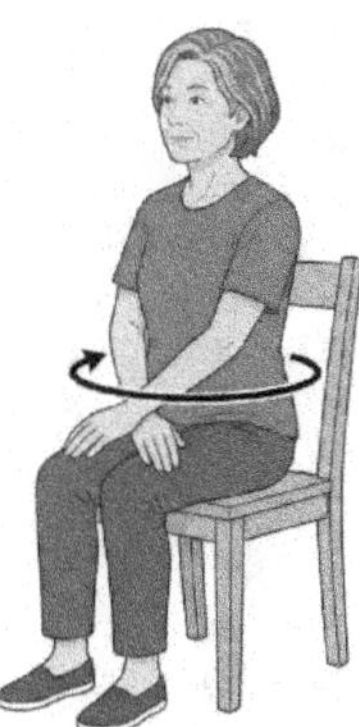

3. Hold for two full breaths at the end of the rotation. Do not force the range.

4. Return to center on an inhale. Repeat to the left side.

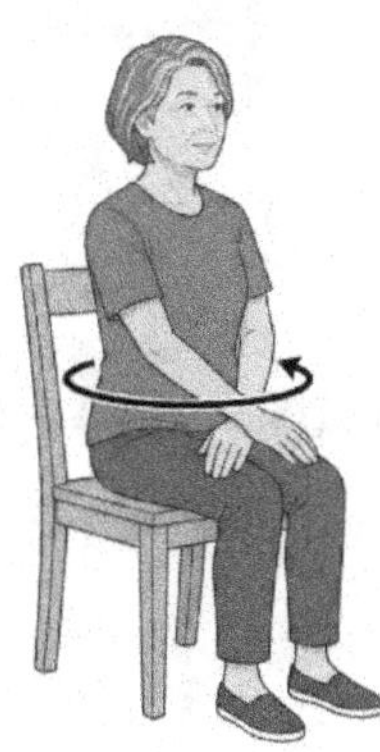

5. Complete three rotations each direction.

BREATHING: Exhale into the rotation. Inhale as you return to center.

FEEL IT: A gentle opening across the mid-back and between the shoulder blades on the rotation side.

IF NEEDED: Reduce the degree of rotation if lower back discomfort occurs. Even a small rotation activates the deep waist muscles.

Micro-Movement 2 – Overhead Arm Press

Decompresses the spine and maintains shoulder elevation range between sessions.

Starting Position:

Sit in Tai Chi neutral, both hands in the lap.

Steps:

1. Interlace the fingers loosely in front of the lower abdomen, palms facing upward.
2. On a slow inhale, raise both arms upward along the centerline of the body, palms turning to face the ceiling as the arms reach overhead.

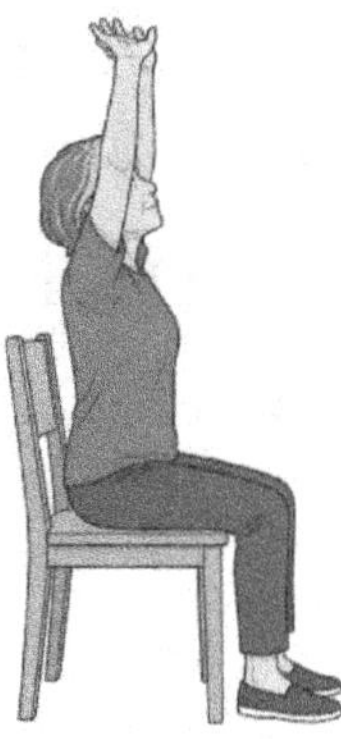

3. At full reach, press the palms gently upward for two counts. Feel the spine lengthen.
4. On a slow exhale, separate the hands and lower the arms in a wide arc back to the lap.
5. Complete five repetitions.

BREATHING: Inhale on the rise. Exhale on the descent.

FEEL IT: A clear decompression in the lower back at full reach. The ribcage expands on the overhead inhale in a way that the chest-only breath does not produce.

IF NEEDED: If overhead reach is restricted at the shoulder, raise the arms to forehead height rather than full extension. The spinal decompression benefit is preserved.

Micro-Movement 3 – Hip Flexor Release

Counteracts the hip flexor shortening that extended sitting produces, restoring the hip extension range that walking depends on.

Starting Position:

Sit at the very front edge of the chair seat, right leg extending back so the right foot is behind the level of the chair front legs.

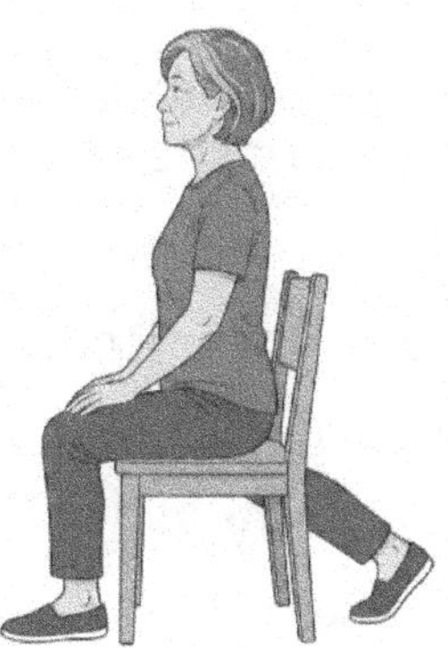

Steps:

1. Sit tall, spine long. The right hip should feel a gentle stretch at the front from the extended leg position.

2. On a slow inhale, lift the right heel slightly off the floor without moving the right knee. Hold two counts.

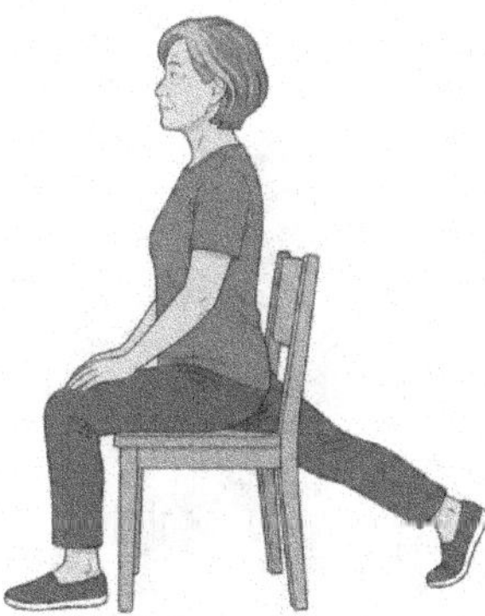

3. On the exhale, lower the heel and slightly deepen the forward lean of the spine from the hips, not the waist, to increase the hip stretch gently.

4. Hold for three full breaths. Return the right foot to a neutral position and repeat on the left side.

5. Complete two repetitions each side.

BREATHING: Breathe into the stretch. Slow steady breath throughout.

FEEL IT: A gentle pull at the very front of the hip crease on the extended side. If this is not present, slide the foot slightly further behind the chair.

IF NEEDED: If sitting at the chair edge is unstable, perform this movement with both feet on the floor by simply rotating the pelvis to a slight anterior tilt and holding for several breaths. Less intense but beneficial.

Micro-Movement 4 – Neck and Shoulder Release

Addresses the postural tension that accumulates at the base of the skull and across the upper trapezius during any sustained seated activity.

Starting Position:

Sit in Tai Chi neutral, both hands resting in the lap.

Steps:

1. Drop the chin slowly toward the chest. Feel the stretch along the back of the neck. Hold two counts.

2. Lift the chin to level. Tilt the right ear toward the right shoulder, a lateral tilt, not a rotation. Left shoulder stays relaxed and down.

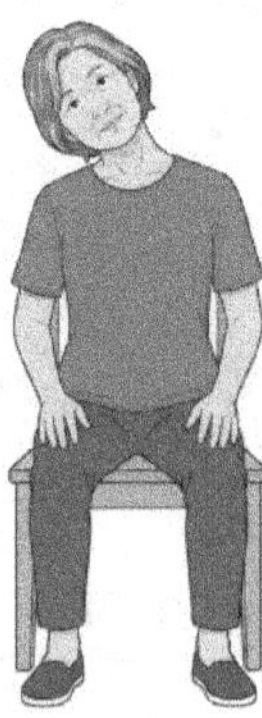

3. Hold three counts. Return to center. Repeat to the left.

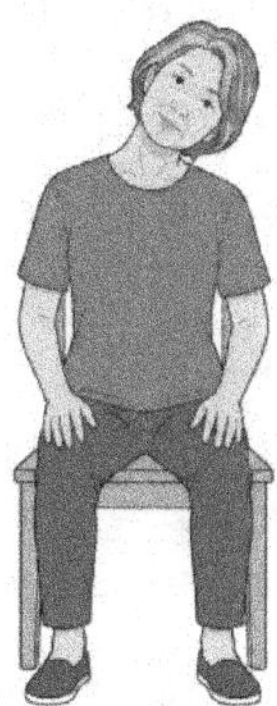

4. Return to center. Perform five slow shoulder rolls backward: up, back, down. Deliberate and full.

5. Let the shoulders settle. They should feel notably lower than when you began.

BREATHING: Inhale as shoulders rise. Exhale as they roll down and back.

FEEL IT: A release of tension across the top of the shoulders and the upper back after the rolls. Many people carry most of their held tension here.

IF NEEDED: If the lateral neck tilt produces discomfort rather than stretch, skip it and perform the shoulder rolls alone. Same upper-back benefit.

> **Jing's Note:** *These four movements exist because the body does not save its improvements for the practice. It uses them continuously. The hip mobility built in Dragon Stirs the Waters matters when you walk to the kitchen and when you step off a kerb. The shoulder range built in Lotus Arms matters when you reach for something on a shelf. Keeping the joints moving between sessions maintains what the practice builds.*

Posture, Core, and Joint Protection

The Tai Chi neutral seated position is the foundation of every form in Chapter Four. It is also the posture that protects the spine, the hips, and the shoulder joints during every moment of daily seated activity. Understanding what it is actually doing makes it easier to apply it beyond the practice chair.

For the lower back:

The natural lumbar curve maintained in Tai Chi neutral distributes load across the intervertebral discs evenly. When the pelvis tips backward and the lower back rounds, the posterior disc surfaces receive disproportionate load. Over hours of sitting this produces the familiar lower back fatigue and discomfort that most people attribute simply to sitting rather than to the specific posture. Maintaining the neutral curve, even partially, throughout the day significantly reduces this load. The practice makes this easier because the muscles that support the curve become progressively stronger.

For the hips:

The soft isometric engagement of the hip muscles in every seated form maintains the health of the hip joint capsule and reduces the compression that sustained passive sitting produces. People who practice Tai Chi consistently often find that the particular ache that develops after 90 minutes in a car seat takes longer to appear and resolves more quickly when it does. This is the hip capsule benefit of regular deliberate hip movement.

For the shoulders:

Maintaining the back-and-down shoulder position throughout the day, not only in the practice, keeps the subacromial space open and reduces the rotator cuff impingement risk that forward-rounded shoulders produce.

Moving Better in Real Life

People come to the practice hoping for weight loss and find that the first clear change is in how they move. They stepped down off a kerb without pausing to prepare. They reached something overhead without the shoulder complaint they had been quietly managing. They got up from a chair in front of others without the small ritual of bracing first.

That is the mobility benefit, and it is not secondary to the weight loss benefit. For most people at this stage, the quality and ease of daily movement matters more than the number on the scale. The practice delivers both, in the order the body is ready for them.

Chapter 8

Life After Day 28

The program is finished. Before you decide what comes next, read this chapter. It will help you read your own results clearly and give you a map of where the practice can go from here.

Taking Stock

There are three broad outcomes that 28 days of consistent seated practice tends to produce, and all of them are real results. The mistake is measuring only one of them and concluding the others did not occur.

Scenario one: exceeded expectations.

Some people feel genuinely different by Day 28. Better sleep, clearly reduced stiffness, more energy in the morning, visible changes in how they sit and move. Some notice the scale has moved. This scenario is common in people who were significantly deconditioned before starting, because their starting point meant the gains of consistent movement were large relative to their baseline. If this is your scenario, the instruction is simple: keep going. You have found the approach that works for your body and your life.

Scenario two: modest progress.

For many people, Day 28 looks something like this: sleep is quietly better, though not dramatically. The morning stiffness that used to take until mid-morning to clear is resolving in twenty minutes. Energy is a bit steadier through the day. The scale has not moved much, if at all. This is actually the most common result and it is a good one. These are not consolation prizes. They are the real changes the first 28 days are designed to produce. The fat loss, the body composition shift, the more visible results: those come from continuing what has already been started. The practice is working. The compounding effect of the next 60 days is where the visible results tend to arrive. Keep going.

Scenario three: minimal change.

A small number of people reach Day 28 and feel that little has changed. Before concluding the practice did not work, it is worth examining a few variables honestly. How many of the 28 sessions were actually completed? Five skipped sessions across a 28-day program is a different program than 28 consecutive ones. Was sleep consistently under six hours? That single variable, if true, could prevent most of the cortisol and metabolic benefits from accumulating. Were food patterns working significantly against the practice? Addressing any one of these variables in a second 28-day attempt typically produces a substantially different outcome.

One thing is worth noting regardless of scenario: the changes that 28 days produces are not erased when the program ends. The neural patterns for the forms are established in the motor cortex. The cortisol baseline has shifted, at least partially. The postural muscles are stronger than they were. The body does not reset when the program finishes. It holds what the practice built, and it builds further if the practice continues.

Whatever your scenario, the assessment is not the end of the story. It is the beginning of an informed decision about the next chapter of the practice.

When the Program Ends But the Practice Doesn't

The 28-day program was a structure for learning the forms and building the daily habit. Now that the forms are in the body and the habit is established, the structure is no longer necessary. What comes next is the practice itself, in whatever form suits your life.

Option A: repeat the program.

Running the 28-day program again is a valid choice, particularly if the first round was interrupted by illness, travel, or irregular sessions. The second run through the program feels qualitatively different. The forms are familiar, which means the attention that was previously occupied with learning can now go to the quality of the movement. Most people who do a second round find that the results are more pronounced, because they arrive at Week Three with a body that has already been preparing for three weeks rather than starting from scratch.

Option B: build your own daily practice.

Use the eight forms and three Circulation Builders from Chapter Four as your daily library. Choose what to include based on how the body feels. A minimum practice on a low-energy day: Breathing Practice, Seated Cloud Hands, Dragon Stirs the Waters, Seated Closing Form. Four minutes. That is still a practice. A full practice: all eight forms, both Circulation Builders, 20 minutes. Most days will fall somewhere between.

The principle is that the practice continues in some form every day, regardless of how much time is available. The minimum version is always better than no version. The habit is maintained by the minimum version even when the full version is not possible. Do not wait for a perfect morning. There is no such thing.

If the idea of choosing your own daily sequence feels daunting, return to Week One of the program and use it as your template indefinitely. Forms 1, 2, and 3, ten minutes. That is a complete practice. It produces all of the core benefits. The more elaborate sequences of Weeks Three and Four build on this foundation but do not replace it. Some practitioners cycle between a simple form and a full one, using the simple version on difficult days and the full version when time and energy allow. Both count.

Adjusting When Results Are Slower

If your Day 28 assessment showed less progress than you expected, the following adjustments are specific and worth attempting in the next 28-day period, addressed one at a time.

If sleep was under six hours consistently:

If your sleep has been consistently short during the program, this is the adjustment most likely to change your next 28 days. Sleep is not passive recovery, it is where the hormonal shifts the practice is building actually complete. No other single change will do more for your results. Three things that tend to help: a fixed wake-up time (even on weekends), a room that is cool rather than warm, and avoiding screens for the 45 minutes before you try to sleep. You can also use the Breathing practice itself as a sleep tool — six cycles of belly breathing in a dark, quiet room activates the same parasympathetic response that makes Tai Chi effective. Let it carry you toward sleep.

If sessions were frequently skipped:

Build the session into a time of day that already has a consistent anchor: the morning before anything else begins, the midday break before eating, the early evening before dinner. The session is most likely to happen when it is attached to an existing habit rather than scheduled as a standalone commitment that competes with everything else. Make the barrier as low as possible. The chair should be in the same place every day. The commitment should be to the minimum version, three minutes if necessary, not the full version or nothing.

If food patterns were working against the practice:

Chapter Six's recommendations are cumulative. Adding protein to one meal is a smaller change than overhauling three meals simultaneously, and it is far more likely to happen and sustain. Start with breakfast. Add a protein source that was not there before. Hold that for two weeks before adding anything else. Gradual is durable. Dramatic is temporary.

Patience with the timeline is itself a form of practice. The body does not hurry its adaptations, and neither should the practitioner.

A final note on the timeline. Most people who practice seated Tai Chi consistently for three months report more noticeable changes than at 28 days. Most who continue to six months report changes they did not anticipate at three. The compounding nature of the cortisol reduction, the muscle activation, and the sleep improvement means that each month of continued practice amplifies the months before it. Twenty-eight days is the starting line, not the finishing tape. The people who reach the most visible results are simply the ones who kept going.

Making This Yours

A practice that sticks is one you make your own. The forms in Chapter Four are there to guide you, not to box you in. The longer you practice, the more you will start to notice which forms your body is asking for on any given day. Dragon Stirs the Waters on the mornings your hips feel tight and hard to move. Gathering the Sky when your lower back feels squashed and needs to open up. Lotus Arms when your chest feels closed in and your shoulders have been hunched for too long. Over time, this stops feeling like a program you are following and starts feeling like something you reach for because you know it helps.

There is no upper limit to how long a seated Tai Chi practice can continue. The forms do not wear out. The body's capacity to benefit from them does not expire. The research on older adults who maintain consistent Tai Chi practice through their seventies and eighties shows continued improvement in balance, cortisol regulation, sleep quality, and reported wellbeing across decades of practice. The 28-day program opened a door. What is on the other side of it is as long as the practitioner chooses to keep practicing.

The chair is still there. The forms are in your body. Whatever comes next, those two things are true.

One last thing worth saying: the people who stay with this practice are not the most disciplined or the most motivated. They are the ones who notice what it does for them and decide it is worth ten minutes. If you are one of those people, the next session is already waiting.

Did You Find This Book Quite Helpful?

If it did, then that's worth something and deserves a place on Amazon.

Leaving a review takes two minutes and nothing else. For a book like this one, written without a publisher's marketing team or advertising spend, that two minutes is how it finds its next reader. It is how someone's daughter spots it while looking for something to give her mother. It is how this work keeps going. Two sentences is all it needs.

Search ***Chair Tai Chi for Weight Loss by Jing Weston*** on Amazon. One or two honest sentences is all it takes.

Thank you for reading. It was an honor to take this trip with you.

Conclusion

When people hear that a movement practice is done entirely from a chair, the first assumption is usually that something has been given up. That the chair is a substitute for the real thing. A concession to a body that cannot do what it used to. This assumption runs so deep in how most people think about exercise that it is worth addressing directly, not in a footnote but here, at the close of the book.

I have watched this assumption erode, session by session, in everyone who has practiced this way consistently. The chair is not a lesser version of the practice. It is the practice, designed specifically for the body that uses it. The forms in this book were chosen and adapted to produce the full range of Tai Chi's physiological benefits from the seated position. The cortisol reduction through diaphragmatic breathing is complete from a chair. The muscle activation that preserves resting metabolic rate is complete from a chair. The joint lubrication, the circulation improvement, the postural muscle strengthening, the proprioceptive training: all of it is available without standing.

What the chair changes is the mechanical environment. What it does not change, in any meaningful sense, is the physiology.

The physical evidence for this is in what the practice produces: measurable cortisol reduction, documented improvement in balance and joint range, preserved and gradually rebuilt muscle tissue, improved sleep quality. These outcomes have been studied in seated Tai Chi populations. They are not theoretical.

The eight forms in Chapter Four were chosen because they produce the specific joint movement, muscle activation, and breath coordination the seated body needs, in a format that can be practiced safely and independently for as long as the practitioner chooses to continue.

What This Practice Gives Back

The people I have worked with over the years have shown me something I did not truly appreciate until I saw it for myself. When someone who has barely moved in years discovers that ten minutes of sitting and practicing leaves them feeling sharper, less achy, and more comfortable in their own body, something bigger than fitness is happening. They are getting a piece of themselves back. The ability to do something good for their own body, on their own, at home, without needing anyone else.

That is what this practice is really about. Not just losing weight. Not just numbers and hormones. It is about feeling your body move, noticing that it responds, and knowing you did that yourself.

That is what feeling better in the chair means. And feeling better in the chair is not the finish line. It is the starting point. Everything else builds from there.

A Final Word from the Author

Sit up straight for a moment. Feel both feet flat on the floor. Let your spine grow a little taller. Take one slow, deep breath from your belly.

That is the whole practice right there. Every form in this book starts and ends exactly like that. You can do it in any chair, in any room, on any day, at any age. You have been doing it for 28 days now. You know how it feels. You know what it does to your body. You know what it changes when you wake up in the morning.

The book is finished. The practice is not. The chair is still there. Sit down tomorrow morning, find the neutral position, take one deliberate belly breath, and begin again. That is all it takes. That is all it has ever taken. The chair was always enough.

About the Author

Jing Weston has practiced Tai Chi for more than two decades and has spent most of that time working with older adults, people managing chronic conditions, and beginners who came to movement late and found it transformed how they lived. He began with group classes at a community center and eventually worked one-on-one with people whose physical constraints required a more individualized approach: patients recovering from joint replacements, people with severe balance deficits, adults in their eighties who had been sedentary for years and wanted to change that.

His teaching approach is grounded in a single conviction: that the body at any age responds to appropriate, consistent movement. Not to dramatic intervention. Not to punishment. To the kind of slow, deliberate, breath-coordinated practice that Tai Chi represents at its core. He has seen this conviction validated too many times to hold it lightly.

He holds decades of attention to how older bodies move, what helps them, and what does not. This book is an attempt to make that attention available to people who cannot be in the same room with him.

He lives simply and practices every morning, usually before the day has fully started.